SURFACE ANATOMY

THE ANATOMICAL BASIS OF CLINICAL EXAMINATION

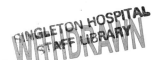

JOHN S.P. LUMLEY

MS FRCS DMCC FMAA(Hon) FGA

Professor of Vascular Surgery, University of London
Civilian Consultant to the Royal Navy in Vascular Surgery
Honorary Consultant Surgeon, St Bartholomew's Hospital, London

Photography by
Carole Reeves
Christopher Priest

Illustrations by
Ian Ramsden

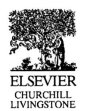

ELSEVIER
CHURCHILL
LIVINGSTONE

EDINBURGH LONDON NEW YORK OXFORD PHILADELPHIA ST LOUIS SYDNEY TORONTO 2002

CHURCHILL LIVINGSTONE
An imprint of Elsevier Limited

First edition 1990
Second edition 1996
Third edition 2002

ISBN 0 443 07045 8
    Reprinted 2002, 2003, 2004, 2005, 2006

International Student Edition ISBN 0 443 07046 6
    Reprinted 2002, 2006

British Library Cataloguing in Publication Data
A catalogue record for this book is available from the British Library

Library of Congress Cataloguing in Publication Data
A catalogue record for this book is available from the Library of Congress

Note
Medical knowledge is constantly changing. As new information becomes available, changes in treatment, procedures, equipment and the use of drugs become necessary. The author, contributor and the publishers have, as far as it is possible, taken care to ensure that the information given in this text is accurate and up to date. However, readers are strongly advised to confirm that the information, especially with regard to drug usage, complies with the latest legislation and standards of practice.

The Publisher

ELSEVIER your source for books, journals and multimedia in the health sciences
www.elsevierhealth.com

Working together to grow
libraries in developing countries
www.elsevier.com | www.bookaid.org | www.sabre.org

ELSEVIER   BOOK AID International   Sabre Foundation

Printed in China
C/06/03

This book describes the visible and palpable anatomy that forms the basis of clinical examination. It should be supplemented by self examination and the examination of normal subjects; and lead to the examination of patients. Students and other models used in practical sessions should come prepared with appropriate clothing, such as swim-wear, and there should be skin pencils and tape measures to hand. In these sessions, a bony skeleton, anatomical models and radiological material should be available for comparison.

The first chapter considers the anatomical terms needed for precise description of the parts of the body and movements from the anatomical positions. There follows a description of pathological terms, clinical examination and the additional tools used in clinical practice.

The remaining chapters are regionally organised and colour photographs demonstrate visible anatomy. Many of the photographs are reproduced with numbered overlays, indicating structures that can be seen, felt, moved or listened to. The surface markings of deeper structures are indicated together with common sites for injection of local anaesthetic, accessing blood vessels, biopsying organs and making incisions. The text describes the anatomical features of the illustrated structures.

The first edition of this text was principally for medical students. However, in subsequent editions, new material has been included to satisfy the needs of other specialties, such as physiotherapy, osteopathy and chiropody. In the present edition, bony attachments and details of joints have been added, and radiological imaging introduced, with radiographs of the skull, chest, abdomen and joints. Information on the spine has been increased and placed in a separate chapter. A new chapter has been added on acupuncture.

London 2002   J.S.P.L.

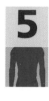

1 INTRODUCTION

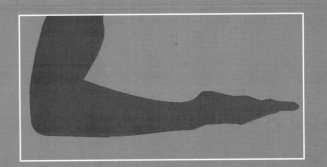

ment is abduction and movement towards the midline is adduction. In

1

ANATOMICAL POSITION

The anatomical position, about which anatomical relationships are orientated, is one in which the subject stands upright, with feet together, eyes looking forward and arms straight down by the sides of the body with palms facing forward (Fig. 1.1). The structures in front are termed anterior (ventral), those behind posterior (dorsal). An exception to this rule is the foot, which is rotated inwards during development: the under (plantar) surface is referred to as ventral and the upper as dorsal. Structures may be nearer (medial) or further from (lateral) the midline and those in the midline are called median. Structures above are superior (cranial, rostral) and those below are inferior (caudal). A sagittal plane passes vertically, anteroposteriorly through the body (the midsagittal plane being in the midline). A coronal plane passes vertically at right angles to the sagittal plane. Transverse (horizontal) planes pass horizontally through the body. Proximal and distal are terms indicating the proximity of a structure to the centre of the body; the wrist is proximal to the hand and the ankle is distal to the knee.

Movement (Figs 1.2–1.8)

Forward movement in a sagittal plane is usually flexion and backward movement extension. Owing to the rotation of the lower limb during development, backward movement of the leg extends the hip and flexes the knee. Upward movement of the ankle is dorsiflexion (extension) and downward movement is plantarflexion (flexion). Downward movement of the toes is flexion.

Movement away from the midline in the coronal plane is abduction and movement towards the midline is adduction. In the case of the digits (excluding the thumb), however, abduction is away from the central line of the middle finger or second toe and adduction is towards it.

Note that the functional axis of the foot is the centreline of the *second* toe.

The thumb is regarded as 'rotated' through 90° with respect to digits 2–5, i.e. its nail faces laterally. Thus extension is lateral

1.1
Anatomical position
A, anterior aspect; B, lateral aspect; C, transverse plane;
D, sagittal plane; E, coronal plane; F, median line

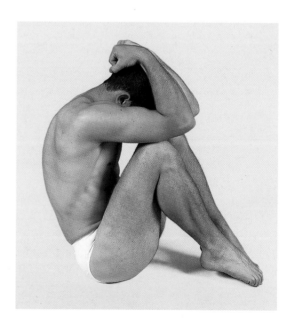

1.2
Flexion

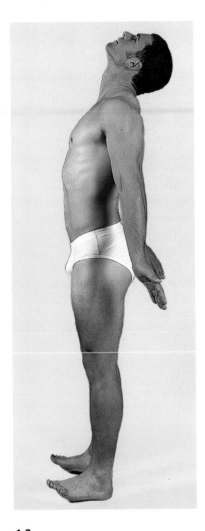

1.3
Extension

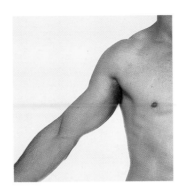

1.4
Abduction

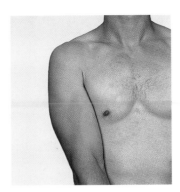

1.5
Adduction

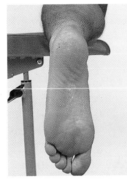

1.6A
Medial rotation

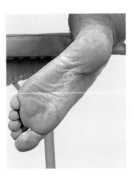

1.6B
Lateral rotation

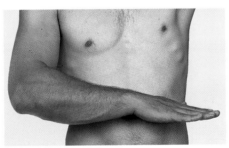

1.7
Pronation

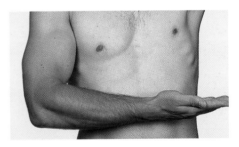

1.8
Supination

movement in the plane of the palm (coronal); flexion is medial movement across the palm; abduction is movement in the sagittal plane (90° to the palmar plane); adduction is return from the abducted position; and opposition is a combination of the above movements with medial rotation. (This also applies to the little finger – Fig. 7.57, p. 86.)

Side-to-side movement of the neck and trunk is termed lateral flexion. Circumduction is the movement when the distal end of a bone describes the base of a cone whose apex is at the proximal end.

Rotation occurs in the long axis of the bone. In the limbs it may be medial, towards the midline, or lateral, away from it. In the upper limb, medial rotation of the forearm is termed pronation and lateral rotation (from the prone to the anatomical position) is termed supination. Turning the sole of the foot towards the midline is termed inversion and away from the midline eversion.

1

PATHOLOGICAL TERMS

This text demonstrates normal anatomy, but abnormal features which are commonly encountered in clinical practice are noted. The pathological terms considered in this section are subsequently used without definition. The study of abnormal (diseased) tissue is termed pathology. Pathologists examine tissues directly by eye (macroscopically), such as in the postmortem room and tissues removed at surgery, or microscopically, when small samples of tissue are specially prepared and looked at under a microscope. Diseases can be classified by their cause and each disease has characteristic clinical and pathological features.

Congenital disease indicates that the abnormality is present before or at birth, although occasionally it does not become apparent until later life. There is sometimes a familial tendency in a number of disease processes and they are then also termed *hereditary*. *Trauma* usually indicates physical violence, with a blunt or sharp instrument. It may also be due to raised or lowered temperature, irradiation, chemicals and the ingestion of poisons. Severe trauma may break bones (fractures) and displace articular surfaces of joints (dislocation). Penetrating wounds (e.g. from a knife or bullet) may damage deep organs, vessels and nerves.

Inflammation is the body's cellular response to injury. It usually occurs against harmful bacteria or viruses, which is termed infection, but also occurs around sites of trauma and around malignant tumours. Cells may reproduce without a stimulus such as infection and form an abnormal mass of tissue known as a tumour or *neoplasm* (the process being neoplasia). This mass may be slow-growing and well circumscribed and is termed a *benign* tumour. Rapidly enlarging tumours growing into adjacent structures are termed *malignant*. Carcinoma is a malignancy of epithelial tissue, but the term is often used as a synonym for any malignancy. Bits of malignant tumour may break off and be carried along lymph and blood vessels to start growing elsewhere. These additional growths are termed secondaries or *metastases*. Secondary growths often occur in lymph nodes; specific sites for lymph node metastases are mentioned in the text. As the body grows older it functions less efficiently and specific *degenerative* diseases can occur such as dementia, with loss of cerebral cells, and hardening and blocking of the arteries (arteriosclerosis). Malfunction of *metabolic* processes and *endocrine* function may produce detectable physical, as well as biochemical, abnormalities.

ANATOMY AND CLINICAL PRACTICE

In clinical practice, clinicians examine living anatomy, and surface anatomy may be the only anatomy encountered in many professional practices. However, all doctors and other clinical professionals need to know the range of normal anatomy, to be able to identify bony and prominent structures, and to know the position of deeply related structures. Superficial and deep tenderness may accompany inflammation and abnormal lumps may be congenital abnormalities, or benign or malignant tumours. Pain and tenderness accompany trauma, and bones and joints are palpated for fractures and dislocations, and deeper relations considered, particularly after penetrating injuries.

Clinical assessment
Examination of the adult patient requires the patient's consent. In the clinical setting, this usually follows *taking a history* of the patient's present and past illnesses and general health. It requires an explanation of what is proposed, and the patient's verbal acceptance. For more invasive procedures, including all surgical operations, written consent must be obtained.

The *clinical examination* must be undertaken in an organised manner, so that it is comprehensive and reproducible, and of a form that inspires confidence in the patient. It is primarily directed at the current clinical problem, but usually involves a general examination of all systems in order to exclude co-existent, sometimes unexpected, disease.

Clinical (bedside) examination involves assessment of each region of the body by inspection, palpation, percussion and auscultation. To this is added the assessment of active and passive movement of the joints and of neurological function. Inspection requires a warm, appropriate, secluded area so that the region being studied is fully exposed and in optimal lighting. The patient is usually lying on his/her back on a couch and the clinician stands on the right side, having first washed and warmed his/her hands. The skin and contours are examined from different angles to identify superficial structures, abnormal swellings and scars, vascular pulsations and movements, such as those related to respiration, swallowing and coughing.

Palpation of superficial structures delineates their shape, surface and consistency. Bony contours can be examined when they are not covered by prominent muscles or other structures. Some superficial nerves and glands are palpable. Lymph nodes such as those inferior to the angle of the mandible, the groin and in the axilla are often palpable and regular examination of these sites is required to appreciate the range of normality.

Movement against resistance will make a muscle belly more prominent; it will thus be more easily palpable and structures deep to it will become less prominent. A superficial artery is most easily palpated when it can be compressed on an adjacent bony surface. The pulps of two or more fingers are placed together along the line of the artery and the distal finger pressed onto the bone to compress the vessel. The proximal finger (or fingers) resting gently on the skin is then used for palpation. The heartbeat can usually be felt by placing the flat of the right hand on the left anterior chest wall. The flat of the hand will also demonstrate chest movements during respiration. Palpation of the abdomen allows a number of abdominal viscera to be felt.

If the middle finger of the right hand is tapped on a table top, first over the central unsupported area and then over one of its legs, the difference between the hollow and the firmer areas will be both heard and felt. If the palm of the left hand is now placed over the same two areas and the right middle finger is used to tap (staccato fashion) the dorsum of the middle phalanx of the left middle finger, the differences of sound and feel will be magnified. This principle is extended to clinical examination by the process of percussion. The palm of the left hand is placed over a body cavity or organ and tapping is carried out as already described. Air-filled organs such as the lungs and the gut sound more hollow than more solid organs such as the heart and liver. Tapping bony surfaces such as the clavicle and skull vault directly with the middle finger can be used to compare the two sides of the body.

Auscultation is the process of listening over the body. This was originally carried out by applying an ear directly over an area. Development of the stethoscope has simplified the manoeuvre and serves to conduct and localise underlying sounds. These sounds include the closing of heart valves, blood flow in some arteries and the movement of air in the trachea, lungs and gut. The bell of the stethoscope is small enough to give easy access to most areas of the body, but the diaphragm of the stethoscope is better for detecting high-pitched sounds.

Assessment of cranial nerve function includes examination of smell, vision, taste, balance and hearing. Pupillary reflexes are assessed by shining a light in the eye and by observing pupil size on alternating near and far vision. Somatic tactile sensation is assessed by the light touch of a finger or a piece of cotton wool; pain is assessed with a gently applied sterilised pin.

Two-point discrimination can be assessed with a blunt-pointed set of dividers. Appreciation of the two ends as separate points of contact ranges from 3–5 mm on the fingers to 4–5 cm on the back.

Vibration sense is assessed with the footpiece of a vibrating large tuning fork and temperature by comparing the side of the examiner's finger with the cold prong of the tuning fork. In other sensory tests the subject closes his/her eyes while a digit is moved backwards and forwards to assess position sense, or the subject is asked to name figures or numbers which have been gently written out on a limb with a blunt instrument. Motor function is assessed by muscle tone, power, coordination and reflexes, the latter being assessed by gently tapping a tendon with a tendon hammer. Muscle mass is compared and abnormal movements noted. In the assessment of lower limb function, the subject is observed walking and standing on one and on both legs.

Assessment of joints is under the headings of *look, feel, move* and *X-ray*, movements being active, passive and resisted. Initial observations provide information on the gait and posture, and detect pain, disability and deformity, such as malalignment and contractures. *Compare* the two sides of the body; it is helpful to examine the non-symptomatic side first when this is normal. The bones and soft tissues around the joint are palpated; resting the hand over a joint during movement may elicit a soft grating sensation know as crepitus due to irregularity of the bony surfaces. Crepitus is also present between the broken ends of a fractured bone but is painful to elicit and fractures can usually

be recognised by local tenderness and the abnormal shape of a bone. *Active movement* is first carried out by the subject. This indicates any limitation of the range of movement, suggesting discomfort or disability. After this has been observed, and following discussion with the subject, the examiner undertakes *passive movement*. This may reveal rigidity or contracture of the muscles, and fixity or abnormal movement of the joints, due to bony or ligamentous abnormalities. Pain noted in active movement can be confirmed by gentle passive movement in the same plane, and may also be revealed in other directions. In *resisted movement*, the examiner exerts counter-pressure as individual muscles are contracted, in order to assess power, pain and discomfort.

The angles of passive and active movement are measured by eye or with a goniometer and a tape measure is used to compare length and circumference of limbs, the latter being taken at appropriate distances from a bony prominence. The circumference may be affected by trauma, inflammation, tumour or muscle wasting. Although a tape measure should always be available to measure normal and abnormal anatomy, some indication of size can be quickly obtained by comparison with part of the examiner's hand: an adult male thumb is approximately 2.5 cm wide, the thumb to the metacarpophalangeal joint 7.5 cm, and the index finger to this joint 10 cm.

General examination

An examination of a subject in clinical practice commences with observation of general features, gaining an impression of the health of the individual and noting sex, age and physique. This part of the examination is based on examination of the head, neck, hands and feet and the shape of the body, without exposing the trunk. It is followed by regional examination of the subject from the head to the feet. This sequence partly follows the systematic pattern by which the examination is reported, but detailed examination of the nervous system is undertaken as a separate entity, so that sensory and motor function are compared throughout the body. It is important to develop a set routine for a complete examination, incorporating thoroughness and, later, speed of execution.

The general health of the subject is assessed by facies, colour, nutrition, hair distribution and shape. Observe normal and abnormal sexual features, such as muscle and fat distribution, and the features of ageing, such as change of stature and loss of skin elasticity. Obesity is noted and any lax skin indicating recent weight loss. General pallor is related to reduced circulating haemoglobin (anaemia) and is best estimated by gently pulling down the lower eyelid and, by so doing, everting it; the colour of the inside of the lid is then assessed. Yellow pigmentation due to raised circulating bilirubin (jaundice) is assessed by the degree of staining of the white sclera of the eyeball. In this general clinical examination, particular attention is given to the hands: the palms, the nails and the texture of the skin over the dorsum provide evidence of nutritional and other pathological disturbances.

Instruments of clinical examination (Figs 1.9–1.11)

The stethoscope, tape measure, cotton wool, sterile pin, torch, tendon hammer and tuning fork have already been referred to.

1

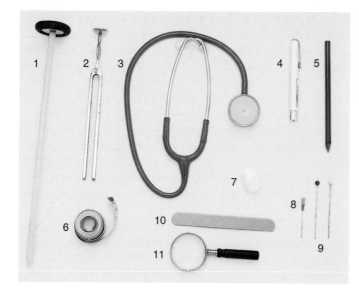

1.9

Instruments of clinical examination
(Disposable gloves are required for oral, rectal and vaginal examination)

1 Patellar hammer
2 Tuning fork
3 Stethoscope
4 Torch
5 Skin pencil
6 Tape measure
7 Cotton wool
8 Sterile needle
9 Red and white headed pins
10 Wooden spatula
11 Magnifying glass

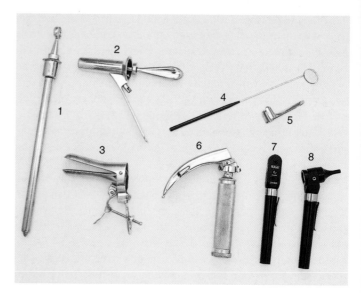

1.10

Speculae and endoscopes

1 Rigid sigmoidoscope
2 Proctoscope
3 Vaginal speculum
4 Laryngeal mirror
5 Nasal speculum
6 Laryngoscope
7 Ophthalmoscope
8 Auroscope

Blood pressure measurement is a routine part of clinical examination. A bandage tied tightly around the upper arm will occlude the brachial artery. If the bell of the stethoscope is placed lightly over the artery distal to this point and the tie gradually released, a pulse is heard as the blood flow is restored. The point at which the sound appears equates to the systolic blood pressure and the point at which the noise suddenly becomes very faint before disappearing, equates to the diastolic blood pressure.

The instrument used to measure blood pressure, the sphygmomanometer, makes use of these principles. A broad, long band of material (the cuff) with an inflatable balloon in its base, is wrapped around the arm. The balloon is attached to a calibrated mercury manometer, so the pressure within it can be measured. After application, the balloon is blown up to a level above the systolic blood pressure, a stethoscope is applied over the brachial artery in the cubital fossa, and the pressure within the balloon slowly released, enabling systolic and diastolic pressures to be measured from the sounds, as already described.

Different cuff sizes are available to measure blood pressure in adults and children. A wider cuff is required for thigh compression, and a Doppler probe to detect the systolic blood pressure, i.e. the point of reappearance of flow when the cuff is deflated.

A number of optical aids have been designed to examine the various recesses, cavities and hollow organs of the body. The ophthalmoscope allows the examination of the retina through the cornea and lens, and the auroscope is designed to view the tympanic membrane. A nasal speculum and a light source allow the examination of the anterior nasal cavities. The mouth is examined

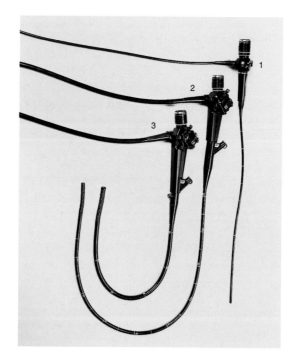

1.11

Fibreoptic endoscopes

1 Bronchoscope
2 Gastroscope
3 Flexible sigmoidoscope

with the aid of a spatula, to depress the tongue, and a torch. A small, angled mirror mounted on a metal rod can be introduced into the oropharynx, without touching its walls, and be turned upwards or downwards to assess the posterior nares or the larynx. The curved lighted smooth metal blade of a laryngoscope allows direct viewing of the larynx, particularly in the anaesthetised patient when the instrument can be used gently to pull the tongue and jaw anteriorly to improve the view.

A large variety of flexible fibreoptic instruments are used to view the interior of the body. A bronchoscope is used to examine the larynx, trachea and main bronchi. A longer and firmer instrument can be passed along the upper alimentary tract to observe the oesophagus, stomach, duodenum and sphincter of Oddi.

The anal canal, lower rectum and vagina are examined with a gloved finger and through lighted metal tubes (proctoscope, sigmoidoscope, vaginal speculum). The lower alimentary tract can be examined from the anal canal to the ileocaecal valve with a colonoscope. The urethra and bladder can be visualised through flexible or rigid instruments identifying the ureteric orifices, which themselves can be entered by catheters and contrast medium introduced to outline the renal pelvis and ureter. Other fibreoptic instruments can be introduced through small incisions to examine body cavities such as the pleural or peritoneal cavity, and the interior of joints.

Abnormal surface tissue can be sampled (biopsied) and submitted to subsequent pathological examination. A knowledge of the surface markings of the superficial and larger, deep, blood vessels allows the introduction of needles or cannulae to obtain blood samples, measure pressures or introduce radiological contrast medium, fluid requirements and drugs. Needles may also be introduced into a hollow, cystic or solid organ or mass, to inject into them or to obtain fluid or solid biopsy samples. Knowledge of the position and distribution of peripheral nerves allows injection of local anaesthetic to relieve pain or to undertake pain-free operative procedures.

A surgeon requires to know the detailed topographical anatomy of each operation undertaken, but all clinicians should be aware of the common surgical incisions and the likely procedure that has been undertaken through an old operation scar.

Bony structures show up on conventional radiographs and these can be related to examination findings. Injection of radio-opaque material into the bloodstream, body cavities or hollow organs· allows vessels, cavities and organs to be outlined. Scanning apparatus, such as ultrasound, computed tomography (CT) and magnetic resonance imaging (MRI), demonstrate normal and abnormal bone and soft tissues, supporting clinical findings. They may also be used to direct the positioning of needles for sampling or injection. Isotope scans measure radiation from isotopes passing through or accumulating in a specific region, indicating blood flow and metabolic activity.

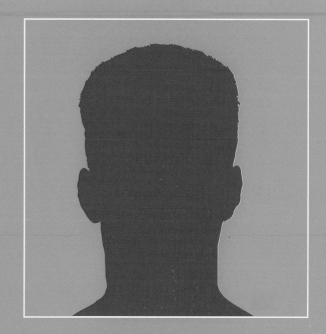

FACE

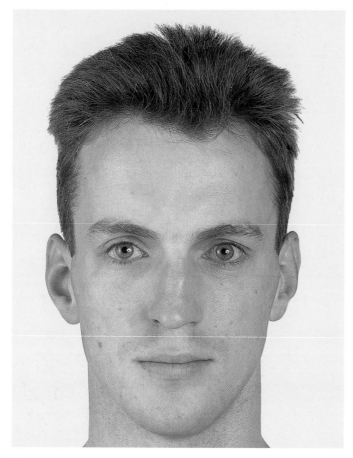

2.1
Anterior aspect of the face

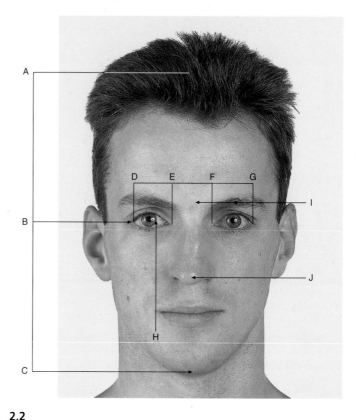

2.2
Facial alignment

A, B, C	In the adult, the eyes are sited halfway between the vertex and the chin, whereas at birth they are at the junction of the middle and lower thirds
D, E, F, G	The eyes are an eye width apart
H	The angle of the mouth is in line with the medial border of the iris
I, J	The tip of the ear is in line with the eyebrow and the glabella, and the lobule is in line with the tip of the nose

Facial bones (Fig. 2.3)

The forehead is formed by the smooth convexity of the frontal bone. The inferior, curved borders of the bone, sharp medially and rounded laterally, form the superior margin of each orbit. The palpable supraorbital notch (or foramen) is sited at the junction of the medial and middle third of each margin; it transmits the supraorbital vessels and nerve, and the artery may be palpable. Medially, above the orbital margins, are the superciliary arches, which are more prominent in the adult male. The arches are united across the midline by a prominent ridge, the glabella; the depression beneath this is the nasion.

The frontal bone articulates with the frontal process of the maxillary bone along the medial aspect of the orbit and, together with the lacrimal bone, houses the lacrimal drainage apparatus just within the orbit (p. 15).

The two nasal bones articulate with each other, with the frontal bone and with the frontal process of the maxillary bone. The internasal and frontonasal sutures meet at the nasion. The lateral border of the orbit is formed by the frontal and zygomatic bones and the frontozygomatic suture can be palpated along this margin. The zygomatic bone forms the prominence of the cheek and, with the maxillary bone, the inferior margin of the orbit. It has a posterior process which, with the zygomatic process of the temporal bone, forms the zygomatic arch (Fig. 2.15).

The inferior alveolar margin of each maxilla carries the sockets for the teeth and the bone houses the maxillary air sinus. It also forms parts of the lateral wall of the nose and the hard palate (Fig. 2.23). The infraorbital foramen in the maxilla is in line with the supraorbital notch; it is 1 cm below the inferior orbital margin and transmits the infraorbital nerve.

The mandible contains the sockets for the lower teeth. The mental foramen transmits the mental vessels. At birth it is near the inferior margin, but in the adult it is midway between the alveolar and inferior margin of the mandible; it becomes nearer the upper margin with tooth loss and bone resorption.

Facial muscles

The skin around the face is thin, vascular, sensitive and, in the male, hairy with abundant sweat and sebaceous glands. There is a variable amount of fat but no deep fascia. The skin over the nose is adherent to the nasal cartilages but not to the nasal, frontal or maxillary bones. The two nasal cavities are separated by the midline nasal septum and open anteriorly at the anterior

2

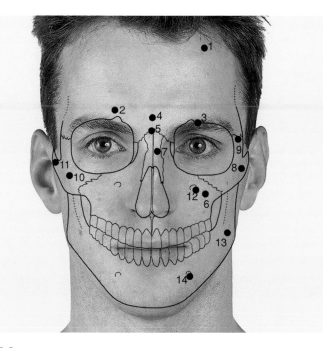

2.3
Anterior aspect of the face: bones

1 Frontal bone	8 Zygomatic bone
2 Superciliary arch	9 Frontozygomatic suture
3 Supraorbital notch	10 Prominence of cheek
4 Glabella	11 Zygomatic arch
5 Nasion	12 Infraorbital foramen
6 Maxilla	13 Mandible
7 Nasal bone	14 Mental foramen

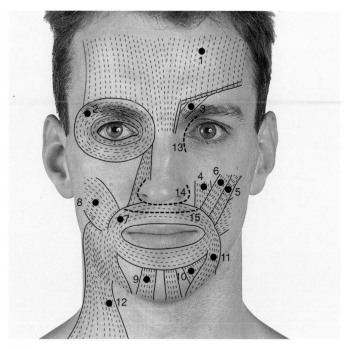

2.5
Anterior aspect of the face: muscles and incisions

1 Frontalis	9 Mentalis
2 Orbicularis oculi	10 Depressor labii inferioris
3 Corrugator	11 Depressor anguli oris
4 Levator labii superioris	12 Platysma
5 Zygomaticus major	13 Medial orbital incision
6 Zygomaticus minor	14 Infranasal incision
7 Orbicularis oris	15 Sublabial incision
8 Buccinator	

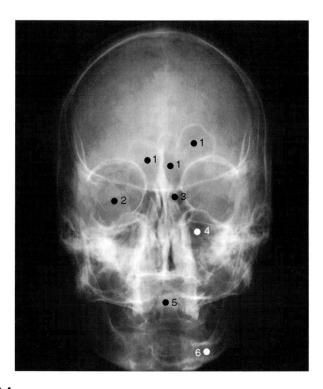

2.4
Skull radiograph: anterior view

1 Frontal air sinus	5 Odontoid process of axis
2 Orbit	vertebra
3 Ethmoidal air sinus	6 Ramus of mandible
4 Maxillary air sinus	

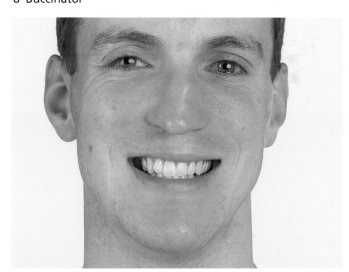

2.6
Muscles are used to produce various facial expressions

nares. Examination of these openings using a torch reveals the wider vestibule within the expanded ala and usually the anterior end of the inferior turbinate bone. The muscles of facial expression are arranged as sphincters and dilators around the orbit, nose and mouth (Fig. 2.5). Their actions are linked with the mood of an individual and they are innervated by the facial (7th cranial) nerve (Fig. 2.6). The frontalis muscle blends with the occipital aponeurosis, and the platysma with the subcutaneous tissue of the neck and upper thorax.

In deep cuts of the face, sutures are placed in the muscles as well as the skin. Incisions follow skin creases, such as around the side and base of the nose and along the medial aspect of the orbit, or are mucosal within a cavity such as the mouth. The three incisions shown in Figure 2.5 can all be used to gain access to the sphenoidal air sinus and the pituitary gland in spite of the depth of the latter structure. A microscope, a strong light and long fine instruments are used.

LATERAL ASPECT OF THE HEAD

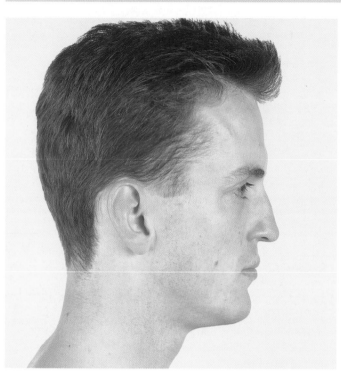

2.7
Lateral aspect of the head

The lateral aspect of the skull vault is formed of the frontal, parietal and occipital bones; the first two meet in the midline at the bregma and the last two at the lambda (Fig. 2.8). These sites are unfused at birth and are known respectively as the anterior and posterior fontanelles. The triangular-shaped posterior fontanelle (lambda) closes 2–3 months after birth and the diamond-shaped anterior (bregma) at approximately 18 months. Four bones (frontal, parietal, greater wing of sphenoid and the squamous temporal bone) meet in H-shaped fashion in the temporal region, overlying the middle meningeal artery; this point is known as the

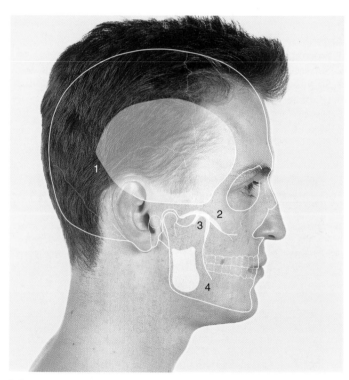

2.9
Lateral aspect of the head: muscle attachments
1 and 3 Temporalis   2 and 4 Masseter

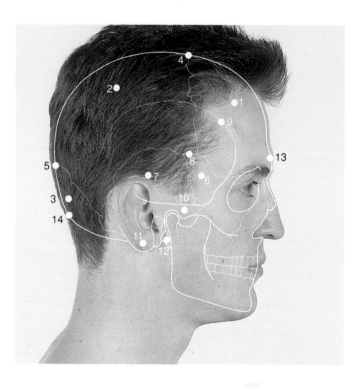

2.8
Lateral aspect of the head: bones

1 Frontal	7 Squamous temporal
2 Parietal	8 Pterion
3 Occipital	9 Temporal line
4 Bregma (anterior fontanelle)	10 Zygomatic arch
5 Lambda (posterior fontanelle)	11 Mastoid process
6 Greater wing of sphenoid	12 Styloid process
	13 Glabella
	14 Inion

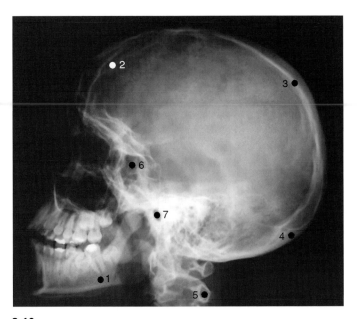

2.10
Skull radiograph: lateral view

1 Mandible
2 Frontal bone
3 Parietal bone
4 External occipital protuberance
5 Spine of second cervical vertebra
6 Sphenoidal air sinus
7 External auditory meatus

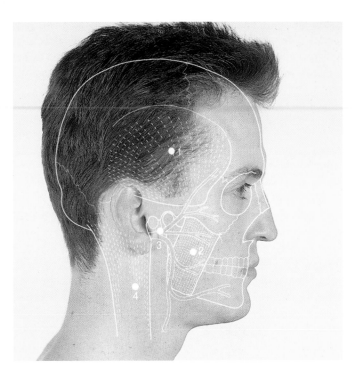

2.12
Lateral aspect of the head: soft tissues

1 Temporalis muscle
2 Masseter muscle
3 Divisions of the facial nerve
4 Sternocleidomastoid muscle

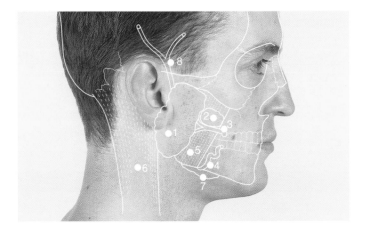

2.11
Parotid gland

1 Parotid gland
2 Accessory lobe
3 Parotid duct
4 Facial artery
5 Masseter muscle
6 Sternocleidomastoid muscle
7 Submandibular gland
8 Superficial temporal artery

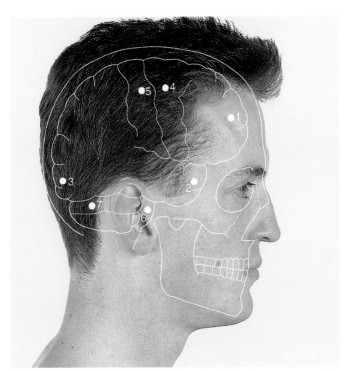

2.13
Lateral aspect of the skull: the surface markings of the brain

1 Frontal pole
2 Temporal pole
3 Occipital pole
4 Precentral gyrus
5 Postcentral gyrus
6 Pons
7 Cerebellum

pterion. A burr hole is placed through the skull at the pterion to evacuate the blood clot when there is uncontrolled haemorrhage from a damaged middle meningeal artery, as in a skull fracture. (The pterion is also called the sylvian point because it overlies the stem of the sylvian, or lateral, cerebral sulcus.)

The processes of the frontal and zygomatic bones, forming the lateral border of the orbit, also form the anterior border of the temporal fossa. The palpable temporal line gives attachment to the temporalis fascia. The temporalis muscle is attached

2

below this line and can be felt when biting (Fig. 2.12); it is supplied by the mandibular nerve. The temporalis fascia is attached inferiorly to the zygomatic arch which is formed by the temporal process of the zygomatic bone and the zygomatic process of the squamous temporal bone.

The masseter muscle passes from the outer posterior inferior aspect of the mandible to the inferior margin of the zygomatic arch. Its shape is accentuated by clenching the teeth, and the facial artery is palpable crossing the inferior margin of the mandible just in front of the anterior border of the muscle. The masseter is supplied by the mandibular nerve.

The parotid gland is wedged between the ramus of the mandible anteriorly, with the masseter superficial and medial pterygoid muscles deep to the bone (Fig. 2.11). Posteriorly is the mastoid process, with the sternocleidomastoid superficial and the posterior belly of the digastric muscle deep to the process. Medially lies the styloid process (Fig. 2.8) with its attached and related structures; superiorly, the cartilaginous external acoustic meatus and the temporomandibular joint. The accessory lobe of the gland lies superficial to the masseter muscle and the parotid duct can be felt passing anteriorly over the contracted muscle. The duct then turns medially to pierce the buccinator muscle and open into the vestibule of the mouth opposite the crown of the second upper molar tooth. Swellings in the lower pole of the parotid gland can present just posterior to the angle of the

mandible and may be mistaken for swellings originating in the submandibular region.

Surgical incisions of the skull and parotid gland (Fig. 2.14)

Emergency surgery is sometimes required when fractures across the temporal fossa damage the middle meningeal artery. Blood collects between the bone and the dura and needs to be relieved by removal of some overlying bone. The vertical incision is through the skin and temporalis fascia and muscle. Bone over the pterion is removed, centred 3.5 cm posterior and 1.5 cm above the frontozygomatic suture. Access to the brain can be gained either through a single bony hole, allowing biopsy of the underlying brain, or by raising a flap of bone (craniotomy). The incisions marked indicate common sites for craniotomy, allowing access to different cortical regions.

The surgical approach to the parotid gland follows the anterior border of the auricle and then passes along the upper anterior border of the sternocleidomastoid muscle. The skin and superficial tissues are dissected forward off the gland. The facial nerve passes through the parotid gland but the superficial portion of the gland and its duct can be excised without damaging the nerve, provided it is identified and preserved and the disease for which the operation is being undertaken does not involve the nerve. The nerve can be identified by a nerve stimulator, observing contraction of the appropriate facial muscles.

Temporomandibular joint (Fig. 2.15)

The inferoposterior margin of the zygomatic arch forms the upper articulation for the temporomandibular joint. The body, the angle and the ramus of the mandible are palpable. The condyle of the mandible is the inferior articulation of the

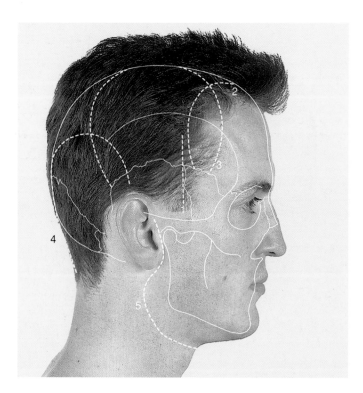

2.14
Surgical incisions of the skull and parotid gland
  1 Surgical approach to the pterion
2–4 Frontal, temporoparietal and occipital craniotomy
       incisions
  5 Incision for surgical approach to the parotid gland

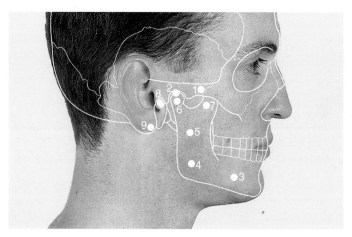

2.15
Temporomandibular joint

1 Zygomatic arch	6 Condyle of mandible
2 Temporomandibular joint	7 Coronoid process of
3 Body of mandible	mandible
4 Angle of mandible	8 External acoustic meatus
5 Ramus of mandible	9 Mastoid process

divided into superior and inferior compartments by a fibrocartilaginous disc that is attached around its perimeter to the joint capsule. The coronoid process of the mandible gives attachment to the temporalis muscle but it lies deep to the zygomatic arch and is impalpable. Movement of the mandible involves both temporomandibular joints. Similar movement occurs in both joints in descent, elevation, protrusion and retraction, but contrary movement is present in the two joints during rotation and grinding. The most powerful movement is elevation, as in the bite; it is produced by the temporalis, masseter and medial pterygoid muscles, while the medial and lateral pterygoid muscles act together in protrusion. Abnormalities of dental occlusion may give rise to pain and stimulate remodelling of the joint articular surfaces. Dislocation of the temporomandibular joints can only take place in an anterior direction, this occurring when trauma is applied to the open mouth.

The external acoustic meatus opens below the posterior end of the zygomatic arch. The palpable mastoid process projects downwards behind the meatus. The superficial temporal artery is palpable as it crosses the zygomatic arch just in front of the external acoustic meatus and its anterior and posterior branches can be traced by palpation over the temporal region.

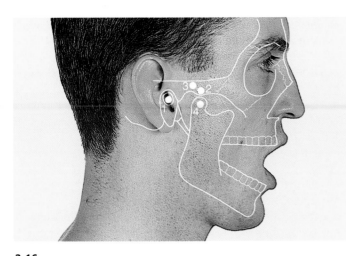

2.16
Opening the jaw
1 External acoustic meatus   3 Zygomatic arch
2 Articular tubercle   4 Condyle of mandible

temporomandibular joint; it is not easily palpable with the jaw closed, because of a prominent lateral ligament, but it becomes so when the jaw is opened and the condyle moves forward on the articular eminence of the joint (Fig. 2.16). The joint is

EYE

The orbit is limited anteriorly by the upper and, smaller, lower eyelids, which are united medially and laterally, limiting the palpebral fissure. Each lid contains a dense fibrous tarsal plate and numerous modified sebaceous (tarsal) glands opening onto the margin behind the eyelashes; the latter are arranged in two or three irregular rows. Medially the eyelids enclose a pinkish elevation, the lacrimal caruncle. An elevation on the medial end of each lid, the lacrimal papilla, has a punctum through which tears are drained into the lacrimal apparatus (Fig. 2.18). The conjunctiva lining the inner aspect of each eyelid is continuous with that over the front of the eyeball. Closure of the eyelids thus produces a sealed cavity into which lacrimal fluid secreted

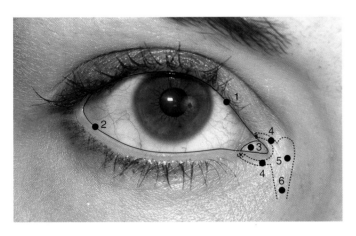

2.17
The eye
1 Upper eyelid   3 Lacrimal caruncle
2 Lower eyelid   4 Lacrimal canaliculi
The opening between the   5 Lacrimal sac
upper and lower lids is the   6 Nasolacrimal duct
palpebral fissure

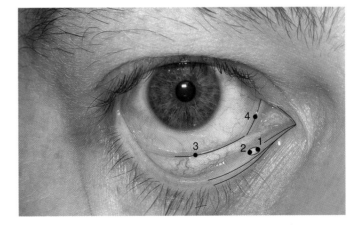

2.18
The eye
The lower lid has been everted to show:
1 Lacrimal papillae   3 Conjunctival fornix
2 Lacrimal punctum   4 Plica semilunaris

2

by the lacrimal gland can circulate, lubricating the conjunctiva and passing medially to drain into the lacrimal apparatus through the lacrimal canaliculi. The eyelids are closed by the orbicularis oculi muscle and the upper lid is raised by levator palpebrae superioris.

The eyeball is embedded in orbital fat. The suspensory ligaments supporting the globe are attached to the medial and lateral margins of the orbit, and the position of the eye is controlled by the extraocular muscles. The anterior segment of each eye opens to the exterior through the palpebral fissure between the eyelids. It is lined by conjunctiva and lubricated by the secretions of the lacrimal gland, passing into the conjuctival sac through approximately 12 ducts under the lateral aspect of the upper lid. The fluid drains through the lacrimal puncta and the nasolacrimal apparatus into the nose, this being facilitated by the muscular action of blinking.

The orbit can be entered for surgery on the eye muscles and abnormalities within the orbital cavity by incision of the conjunctiva along the upper or lower margin of the conjunctival sac (conjunctival fornices).

The extraocular muscles contract and relax in a coordinated fashion, enabling the two eyes to focus on and to follow an object. Looking to the left involves the left lateral rectus muscle, supplied by the abducent (6th cranial) nerve; looking down and to the left involves the left superior oblique muscle supplied by the trochlear (4th cranial) nerve. The other extraocular muscles are supplied by the oculomotor (3rd cranial) nerve.

Abnormalities of gaze may indicate intracranial damage to these cranial nerves or their nuclei (Fig. 2.19).

Touching the cornea with a whisk of cotton wool produces a blink (corneal reflex); shining a bright light into the pupil produces reflex pupillary contraction of both the stimulated and the contralateral eye (pupillary reflex and consensual response). The pupils will also contract when changing focus from a distant to a near object (accommodation reflex).

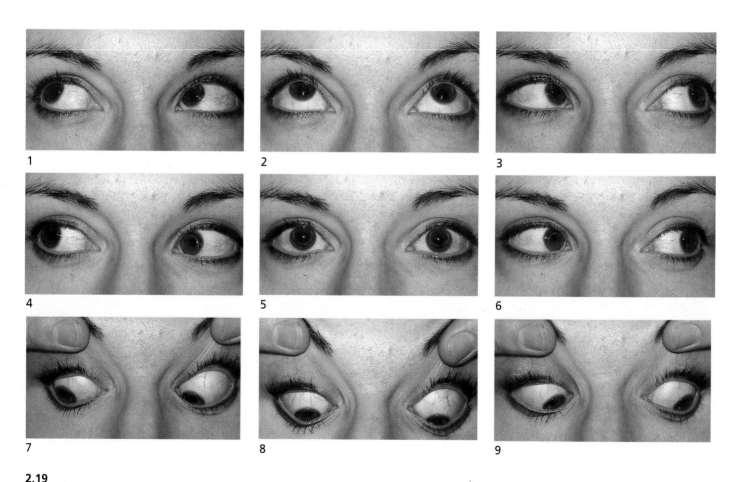

2.19

The nine cardinal positions of gaze

The action of the lateral rectus muscle is seen in the right eye in position 4. The superior oblique muscle, acting independently, depresses the eyeball and is a weak abductor. However, the line of the oblique portion of the muscle is nearest the visual axis in adduction. Thus the maximum depressor effect of the right superior oblique muscle is in position 9. When the right eye is abducted, depression (position 7) is produced primarily by the inferior rectus muscle and the pull of the oblique portion of the superior oblique is at right angles to the visual axis. In this position, the prime action of the superior oblique muscle is in torsion, pulling the top of the eyeball towards the nose.

The pyramidal-shaped external nose has two inferior elipsoid apertures – the nostrils, or external nares, situated behind the tip and separated by the nasal septum. The nose is expanded lateral to each nostril as the ala nasi. Each nostril leads into a nasal cavity that lies alongside the nasal septum. The supporting framework of the nose is made up of the two nasal bones superiorly, and surrounded by the frontal process and body of each maxilla (Fig. 2.3, p. 11). The remaining framework is made up of a series of nasal cartilages. The nose is prone to injury, and although the cartilage usually recoils to its normal position, fracture of the nasal bones may be accompanied by deformity, sometimes requiring refashioning.

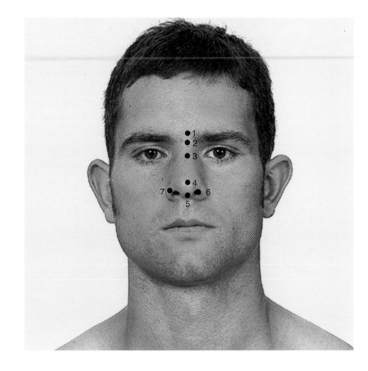

2.20
The nose
1 Glabella
2 Nasion
3 Bridge of nose
4 Tip of nose
5 Nasal septum
6 External nares
7 Ala nasi

The oral cavity is the first part of the alimentary tract and extends from the lips to the isthmus of the fauces. It contains the tongue and alveolar arches with the gums and teeth, and receives the openings of the salivary glands. Its mucous membrane starts on the oral aspect of the lips at the red margin. The alveolar arches and teeth divide the cavity into an outer vestibule and an inner mouth cavity proper. The vestibule is a slit-like cavity when the lips and teeth are opposed, communicating with the mouth cavity behind the molar teeth. The parotid duct opens into

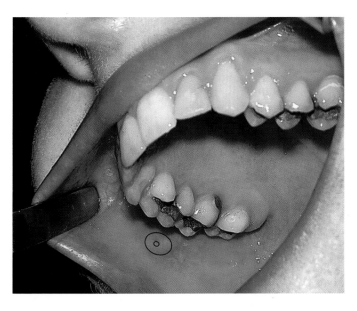

2.21
The vestibule
The opening of the parotid duct is shown opposite the crown of the second upper molar tooth.

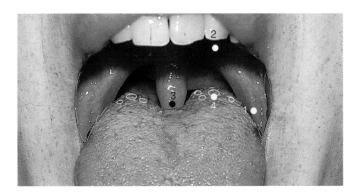

2.22
Soft palate and uvula at rest
1 Anterior arch of the fauces
2 Soft palate
3 Uvula
4 Circumvallate papillae at the junction of the anterior two-thirds and posterior third of the tongue

2

the vestibule just above the crown of the second upper molar tooth (Fig. 2.21). In the mouth cavity proper, the roof is formed by the hard and soft palates, the former being formed by processes from the maxilla and palatine bones. The soft palate ends in the midline posteriorly as the uvula.

The posterior opening of the oral cavity is the faucial isthmus, which is bounded laterally by the palatoglossal fold (the anterior arch of the fauces), superiorly by the soft palate and inferiorly by the tongue (Figs 2.22, 2.23). The palatine tonsil lies behind the fold, between it and the palatopharyngeal fold (the posterior arch of the fauces) (Fig. 2.24).

The tongue lies in the floor of the mouth. A V-shaped sulcus terminalis, with the point posteriorly, divides the anterior two-thirds from the posterior third which has different embryological origins and nerve supply. A midline fold of mucous membrane, the frenulum, connects the undersurface of the tongue to the floor of the mouth. On each side of this is a sublingual papilla onto which opens the submandibular duct (Fig. 2.25). Passing backwards from the papilla on each side sublingual folds of mucous membrane overlie the sublingual glands.

Average eruption time of each half of the upper and lower jaws:

Deciduous teeth

Incisors $\frac{7}{6}\frac{8}{9}$ Canines $\frac{18}{18}$ Molars $\frac{12}{12}\frac{24}{24}$ months

Permanent teeth

Incisors $\frac{7}{7}\frac{8}{8}$ Canines $\frac{12}{12}$ Premolars $\frac{9}{9}\frac{10}{10}$

Molars $\frac{6}{6}\frac{12}{12}\frac{18+}{18+}$ years

The teeth of the upper jaw are innervated by the posterior and superior alveolar nerves; the upper gums, on the labial surface, by the infraorbital and posterior alveolar nerves and, on the lingual surface, by the nasopalatine and greater palatine nerves. Local anaesthesia is usually by injection around the tooth. The lower teeth are supplied by the inferior alveolar nerve, the labial surface of the gums by the mental and buccal nerves, and the lingual surface by the lingual nerve. The incisors are bilaterally innervated and are anaesthetised by injection of local anaesthetic adjacent to the teeth. Injection around the inferior alveolar nerve as it passes to enter its canal, also the adjacent lingual nerve, anaesthetises the lower gums, the teeth and the tongue.

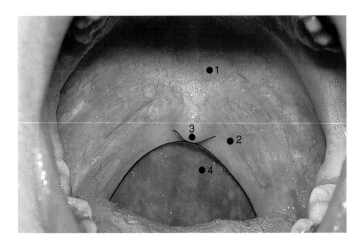

2.23
Soft palate and uvula raised
1 Hard palate   3 Uvula
2 Soft palate   4 Oropharynx

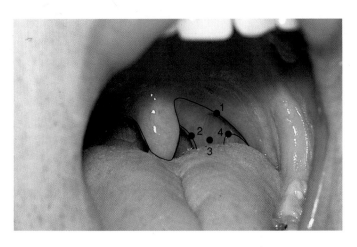

2.24
Palatine tonsil
1 Anterior arch of the fauces   4 Upper border of the
2 Posterior arch of the fauces   palatine tonsil
3 Tonsillar fossa

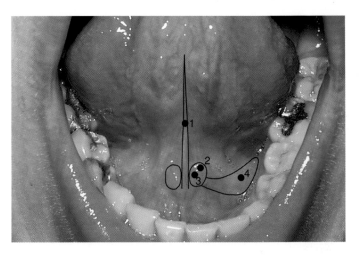

2.25
Under surface of the tongue
1 Frenulum   4 Sublingual fold
2 Submandibular papillae
3 Opening of submandibular
   duct

2

The auricle is a single irregularly shaped piece of elastic cartilage covered by firmly adherent skin. It has a dependent lobule (which lacks cartilage) and an anterior tragus overlapping the opening of the external acoustic meatus. Other parts of the auricle are labelled in Figure 2.26. Three vestigial muscles attached superiorly to the auricle are supplied by the facial nerve. The external acoustic meatus is mainly cartilaginous laterally and bony medially. The tympanic plate of the temporal bone forms the anterior and inferior bony skeleton and the squamous temporal bone, the roof and upper posterior wall. The meatus is approximately 4 cm long and ends medially at the tympanic membrane. It has numerous ceruminous glands in its cutaneous lining and is innervated anteriorly by the auriculotemporal nerve and posteriorly by the vagus (10th cranial) nerve.

The vibration of the tympanic membrane may be inhibited by an excess of wax or by inflammatory changes in the meatus or the middle ear. Inflammation is accompanied by pain and a purulent discharge. Discharge from the meatus is to the exterior. Pus in the middle ear is discharged through the eustachian tube to the nasopharynx, but if this exit is blocked, pus may perforate and discharge through the tympanic membrane.

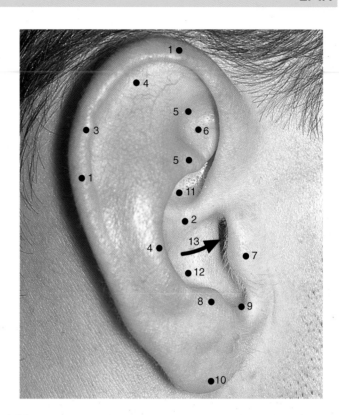

2.26
The ear
1 Helix
2 Crus of helix
3 Auricular tubercle
4 Antihelix
5 Crura of antihelix
6 Triangular fossa
7 Tragus
8 Antitragus
9 Intertragic incisure
10 Lobule
11 and 12 Upper and lower parts of concha
13 Arrow leading to external acoustic meatus

3 NECK

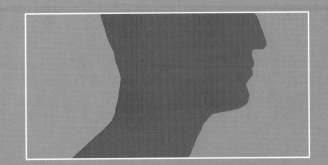

ANTERIOR ASPECT OF THE NECK

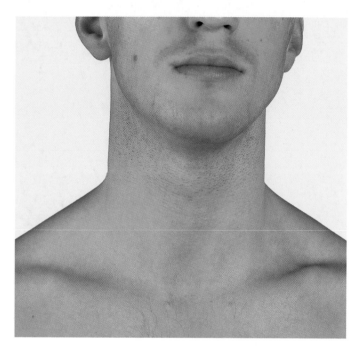

3.1
Anterior aspect of the neck

The anterior aspect of the neck is bounded by the body and angles of the mandible superiorly, and the superior border and sternal notch of the manubrium and the clavicles inferiorly (Fig. 3.2). Laterally it is continuous with the lateral and posterior surface without a specific line of demarcation. The clavicles are subcutaneous throughout their length; they articulate medially at the sternoclavicular and laterally at the acromioclavicular (Fig. 3.11) joints.

Each sternocleidomastoid muscle is attached to the mastoid process and superior nuchal line of the temporal and occipital bones superiorly, and has sternal and clavicular heads inferiorly. The anterior borders of the two muscles form a prominent V shape when contracting together, such as in protruding the chin or raising the head from the lying position. When acting independently, each rotates and laterally flexes the head on the neck, as when looking under a table.

Larynx
The larynx lies in the midline covered only by skin, platysma muscle and superficial and deep fascia. It can be seen to rise during swallowing. Superiorly, the U-shaped hyoid bone is palpable; a central body is bounded laterally by two greater horns (Fig. 3.3). The bone can be gripped between finger and

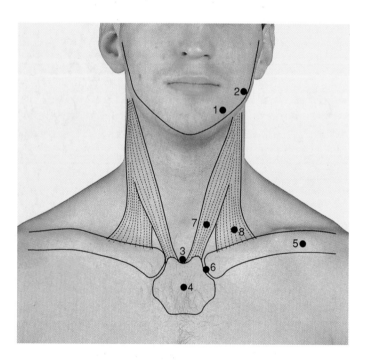

3.2
Anterior aspect of the neck: bones and muscles
1 Body of mandible
2 Angle of mandible
3 Sternal notch
4 Manubrium
5 Clavicle
6 Sternoclavicular joint
7 Sternocleidomastoid muscle – sternal head
8 Sternocleidomastoid muscle – clavicular head

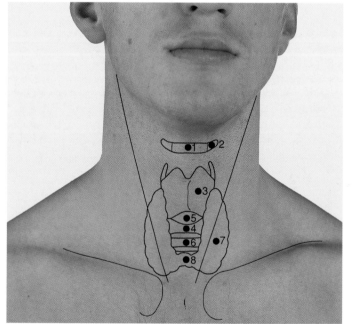

3.3
Larynx and thyroid gland
1 Body of hyoid bone
2 Greater horn of hyoid bone
3 Thyroid cartilage
4 Cricoid cartilage
5 Cricothyroid membrane
6 First tracheal ring
7 Lateral lobe of thyroid gland
8 Isthmus of thyroid gland

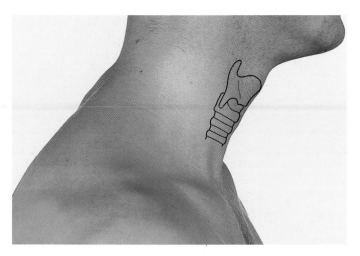

3.4
Laryngeal prominence in the male

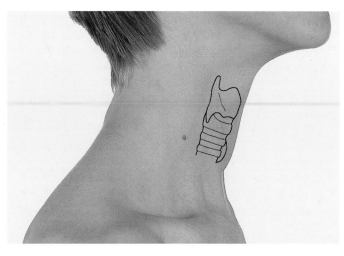

3.5
Laryngeal prominence in the female

3

thumb and if gently pressed backwards and rocked from side to side, the tips of the greater horns can be felt grating against the bodies of the cervical vertebrae, confirming that only thin pre-vertebral muscles and the wall of the pharynx separate the larynx from the vertebral column. The bone is at the level of the third cervical vertebra. Suprahyoid muscles pass to the mandible and into the tongue.

The thyroid cartilage forms a midline prominence which is more obvious in the adult male; the angle between the sides of the cartilage (alae) is approximately 90° in the adult male (the Adam's apple, Fig. 3.4) and 120° in the female (Fig. 3.5). The vocal cords are attached to the back of this prominence, and muscles attached to the oblique line attach the bone to the hyoid superiorly and the back of the manubrium inferiorly. The inferior constrictor muscle of the pharynx is attached to both the thyroid and cricoid cartilages. The latter forms the lower border of the larynx and is the only complete ring of cartilage in the respiratory passage; the adjacent tracheal cartilages are deficient posteriorly. The cricoid and thyroid cartilages are attached anteriorly by the cricothyroid membrane. The lower border of the cricoid is at the level of the sixth cervical vertebra.

Pressure of the cricoid cartilage onto the vertebral column compresses the pharynx, this being a useful manoeuvre to prevent regurgitation of stomach contents into the oropharynx and then into the airway during anaesthesia.

The concept of speech and its use in language is a cortical phenomenon, but its production (phonation) depends on an energy source, a point of vibration and a resonating chamber. The energy is produced by the force of expired air from the lungs and the vibration primarily by the vocal cords. The resonating chamber is the column of air above the vocal cords, including the larynx, pharynx, nasal cavities and mouth.

The primary vowel tones are produced by the sudden opening of the vocal cords during expiration. These glottal sounds are further modified by narrowings in the vocal tract at a higher level, articulating consonants and other sounds – e.g. 'g' and 'k'

by the pharynx and palate; 'd', 's', 'n', 'r' and 'th' by the tongue and teeth; 'f' and 'v' by the lower lip and upper teeth; and 'p', 'b', 'o' and 'oo' by the lips.

Each lateral lobe of the thyroid gland lies adjacent to the thyroid cartilage below the oblique line, overlapped by the strap muscles (omohyoid, sternohyoid and sternothyroid). The lateral lobes are not easily palpable as they are partly covered by the sternocleidomastoid muscles (Fig. 3.3). However, generalised enlargement of the gland (goitre), or a local nodule, is more easily palpable and it is then possible to see the gland moving with the larynx on swallowing. The gland is most easily examined by standing behind a sitting subject. The isthmus of the thyroid gland unites the lateral lobes across the midline anterior to the second and third tracheal cartilages. The first cartilage and isthmus can usually be felt in the midline below the cricoid cartilage. A goitre may be due to iodine deficiency, hormonal imbalance or neoplastic changes within the gland. Surgical access is through a transverse cervical collar incision (Fig. 3.9, p. 25) and care must be taken not to damage the trachea, the recurrent laryngeal nerves or the parathyroid glands.

Anterior triangle (Fig. 3.6)

The sternocleidomastoid muscle divides the anterior and lateral aspects of the neck; the region in front of it on each side is termed the anterior triangle. Two muscles, attached to the hyoid bone (not visible in the living), further divide the anterior triangle into three triangles. The anterior belly of the digastric muscle is attached to the posterior surface of the mandible near the midline and the posterior belly to the mastoid process. The two bellies are joined by an intermediate tendon which is slung to the hyoid bone, and, together with the lower border of the mandible, they form the digastric triangle. The omohyoid muscle passes from the hyoid bone deep to the sternocleidomastoid muscle and, with the anterior border of this muscle and the posterior belly of the digastric muscle, forms the carotid triangle. The muscular triangle is bounded by the omohyoid, the anterior border of sternocleidomastoid, and the midline, from the hyoid bone to the sternum.

A fourth triangle, the submental, crosses the midline; its apex is at the symphysis menti (i.e. the midline bony union of the primitive two halves of the mandible), its lateral margin is the anterior belly of both digastric muscles and its base the body of the hyoid bone.

3.6
Anterior triangle of the neck
The triangle is bordered by the anterior edge of the sternocleidomastoid muscle, the body of the mandible and the midline.

1 Sternocleidomastoid muscle
2 Anterior belly of digastric muscle
3 Posterior belly of digastric muscle
4 Omohyoid muscle
5 Thyroid cartilage
6 Digastric triangle
7 Carotid triangle
8 Cricoid cartilage
9 Muscular triangle

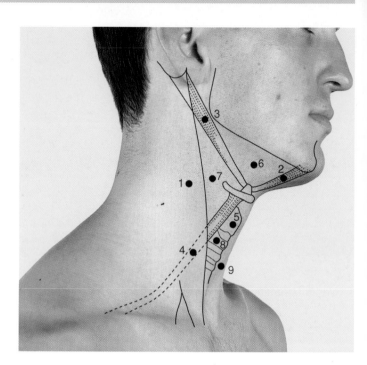

SUBMANDIBULAR REGION

The digastric triangle contains the submandibular gland. The gland lies on and around the posterior border of the mylohyoid muscle, partly overlapped by the body of the mandible just in front of its angle. The facial artery passes over the superior surface of the gland then around the inferior border of the mandible.

The submandibular gland is most easily palpated bimanually, between a finger of one hand placed in the floor of the mouth and the fingers of the second hand placed in the neck over the superficial aspect of the gland. A number of lymph nodes are related to the superficial surface of the gland.

The surgical approach to the submandibular gland is made 2.5 cm below and parallel to the lower border of the mandible in order to avoid the mandibular branch of the facial nerve, which may dip below the mandible as it passes to the lower facial muscles. This incision divides skin, platysma muscle and the superficial and deep fascia, to reach the capsule of the gland and the prominent nodes around it. The same incision can be used to biopsy these nodes or nodes in the carotid triangle.

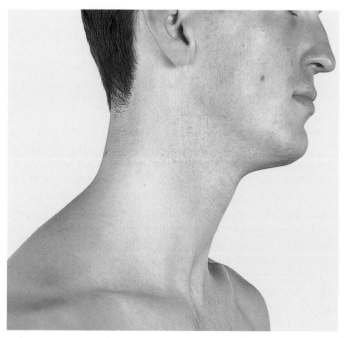

3.7
Submandibular region

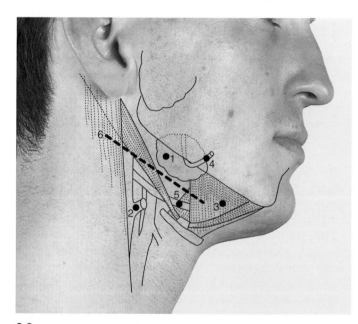

3.8
Submandibular region: soft tissues
1 Submandibular gland
2 Common facial vein
3 Mylohyoid muscle
4 Facial artery
5 Hypoglossal nerve
6 Incision for the surgical approach to the submandibular gland

The larynx is bounded on each side by a cylindrical sheath of fascia (carotid sheath) containing the common carotid artery and the internal jugular vein, and behind these the vagus (10th cranial) nerve; these vessels are covered anteriorly for much of their course by the sternocleidomastoid muscle. The common carotid artery can be palpated above and through the muscle by pressing it posteriorly onto the transverse processes of the cervical vertebrae. It divides at the level of the upper border of the thyroid cartilage into the internal and external carotid arteries. The internal carotid artery passes cranially, with the internal jugular vein, up to and through the base of the skull to supply the brain. The external carotid artery gives branches to the thyroid gland, tongue, face, scalp, pharynx, palate, jaws and nose.

The internal jugular vein lies lateral to the common and internal carotid arteries. In the normal individual, the venous blood pressure is approximately 11 cm above that of the right atrium. By positioning a subject with the upper half of the body raised at an angle of approximately 30° and the head rotated to one side, the characteristic pulse wave of the internal jugular vein can be observed. A needle may be introduced into the common carotid artery for radiological procedures. Access to the internal jugular vein is obtained either superior to the sternocleidomastoid muscle or between its two inferior heads.

The commonest operation in this region is a partial or total removal of the thyroid gland for benign or malignant enlargement. In the collar incision, the skin, platysma muscle and superficial and deep fascia are divided along the line shown (Fig. 3.9). The pretracheal fascia between the strap muscles is divided vertically, or transversely with the strap muscles, to reach the gland; the choice depends on the size and required access to the gland. In diseases of the larynx or in a patient with respiratory difficulty, a temporary or permanent opening may be required into the trachea (tracheostomy). The skin incision may be the central third of the collar incision or a vertical midline approach. The tracheal opening is usually over the second and third tracheal rings and the isthmus of the thyroid gland may also require division. Incision or needle puncture of the cricothyroid membrane enters the larynx below the vocal cords and provides an alternative means of accessing the airway; this is of particular value in children, where the upper trachea is less accessible.

An incision along the anterior border of the sternocleidomastoid muscle through the skin, platysma and superficial and deep fascia, brings the dissection onto the carotid sheath for surgery on the carotid arteries. The upper end of the incision provides access to the submandibular group of lymph nodes (Fig. 3.16). Medial dissection anterior or posterior to the carotid sheath provides access to the pharynx superiorly and the oesophagus inferiorly.

3.9
Carotid arteries, internal jugular vein and applied anatomy
1 Common carotid artery
2 Internal carotid artery
3 External carotid artery
4 Point of access to common carotid artery
5 Internal jugular vein
6 Point of access to internal jugular vein above sternocleidomastoid muscle
7 Point of access to internal jugular vein between the heads of the sternocleidomastoid muscle
8 Collar incision
9 Cricothyroid puncture site

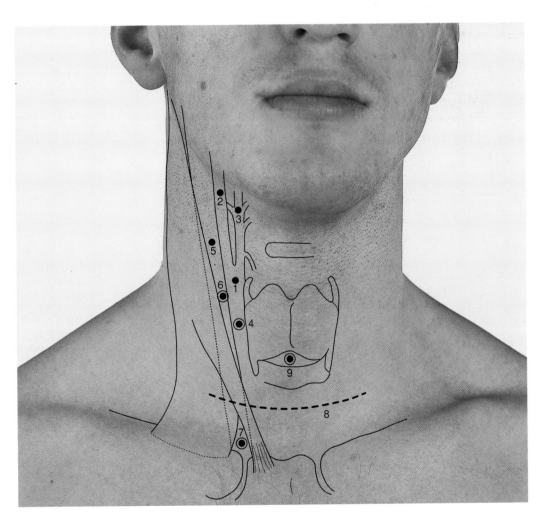

LATERAL ASPECT OF THE NECK

Laterally, the neck is bounded superiorly by the body, the angle and the ramus of the mandible and the temporomandibular joint (Fig. 2.15, p. 14). Behind this are the external acoustic meatus, the mastoid process and the superior nuchal line (Fig. 3.11). The tip of the transverse process of the atlas can be felt by gentle pressure midway between the angle of the mandible and the mastoid process.

Inferiorly, the region is bounded by the clavicle and the acromion which forms the tip of the shoulder. The two bones are united by the acromioclavicular joint.

Posterior triangle (Fig. 3.13)

The posterolateral border of the sternocleidomastoid muscle, with the middle third of the clavicle and the anterior border of the trapezius muscle, form the borders of the posterior triangle of the neck. In a thin subject with the head turned and flexed to the opposite side, the omohyoid can be seen crossing the triangle. The lateral border of scalenus anterior may also be visible. It appears to a variable extent in the anteroinferior angle of the posterior triangle, depending on the size of the clavicular head of the sternocleidomastoid. The apex of the lung rises 3 cm above the medial third of the clavicle. The subclavian artery arches over the lung and the apical pleura behind the scalenus

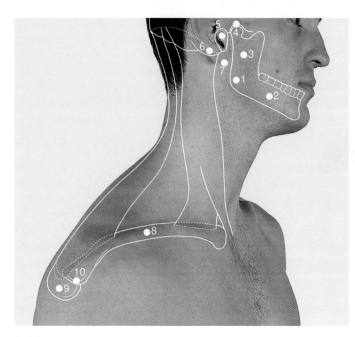

3.11
Lateral aspect of the neck: bones

1 Angle of mandible	7 Tip of transverse process
2 Body of mandible	of atlas
3 Ramus of mandible	8 Clavicle
4 Temporomandibular joint	9 Acromion
5 External acoustic meatus	10 Acromioclavicular joint
6 Mastoid process	

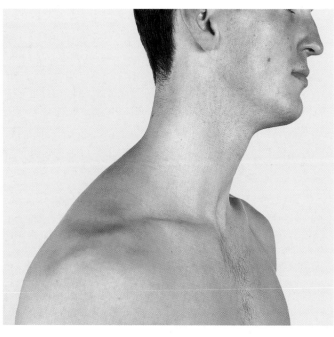

3.10
Lateral aspect of the neek

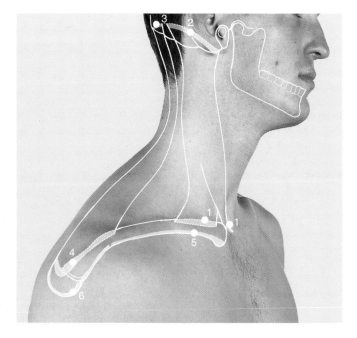

3.12
Lateral aspect of the neck: muscle attachments

1 and 2 Sternocleidomastoid	5 Pectoralis major
3 and 4 Trapezius	6 Deltoid

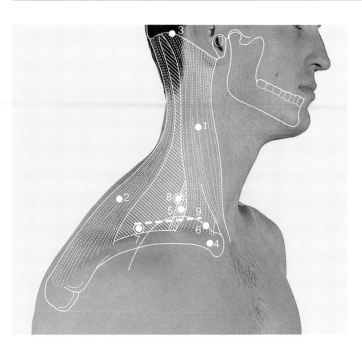

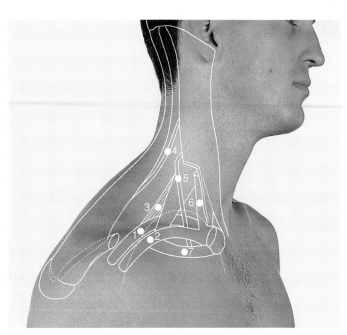

3.13
Posterior triangle of the neck
1 Sternocleidomastoid
 muscle
2 Trapezius muscle
3 Superior nuchal line
4 Clavicle
5 Scalenus anterior
 muscle
6 Apex of lung
7 Needle insertion point for
 brachial plexus anaesthesia
8 Needle insertion point for
 scalene regional anaesthesia
9 Supraclavicular incision to
 approach subclavian artery,
 neck of first rib and
 adjacent structures

3.14
Subclavian vessels and brachial plexus
1 Subclavian artery
2 Subclavian vein
3 Brachial plexus
 (upper trunk)
4 Accessory (11th cranial)
 nerve
5 Phrenic nerve
6 Internal jugular vein
7 First rib

anterior muscle, before passing deep to the clavicle to become the axillary artery and pass through the cervico-axillary canal into the arm (Fig. 3.14). The subclavian artery can be palpated behind the middle of the clavicle by downward pressure onto the first rib.

The subclavian vein lies anterior to the scalenus anterior muscle and is slightly inferior to its artery, being covered by the clavicle.

The vein is frequently used for vascular access. It is usually approached inferiorly but a needle can be inserted into it from above. The point of the needle passes downwards, close to the posterior surface of the clavicle to avoid puncturing the apex of the lung.

The trunks of the brachial plexus may be palpable as they pass obliquely laterally across the anteroinferior angle of the posterior triangle; the lower trunk is, however, deeply placed posterior to the subclavian artery. The trunks divide posterior to the clavicle.

Local anaesthetic can be inserted around the plexus to anaesthetise the arm. A needle is inserted along the lateral border and

deep to the scalenus anterior muscle. More lateral placement of the needle may puncture the apex of the lung.

The accessory (11th cranial) nerve passes anterior to the lateral mass of the atlas and descends through the sternocleidomastoid muscle, then emerging near the middle of the muscle's posterolateral border, it crosses the posterior triangle to reach the trapezius muscle; it supplies both these muscles.

A supraclavicular incision is used to biopsy supraclavicular lymph nodes and to approach the subclavian artery, brachial plexus and cervical sympathetic chain. The last structure is deeply placed across the neck of the first rib. The incision divides the skin, platysma muscle, superficial and deep fascia and the omohyoid muscle. A pad of fat surrounds the omohyoid muscle and encloses the supraclavicular and transverse cervical vessels. The scalenus anterior muscle is divided in line with the incision to reach the subclavian artery and brachial plexus. Care must be taken to preserve the phrenic nerve as it crosses the scalenus anterior muscle and the apex of the lung behind the muscle.

CUTANEOUS INNERVATION OF THE HEAD AND NECK

The trigeminal (5th cranial) nerve supplies the facial area, in front of the thick line shown in Figure 3.15, through its named branches. The remaining cutaneous supply is from the cervical nerves; the dorsal roots innervate the skin posterior to the dotted line. The greater occipital nerve is derived from the second cervical nerve; the first provides motor innervation of the suboccipital muscles but has no cutaneous contribution from its posterior primary rami. The ventral roots, forming the cervical plexus, innervate the skin anterior to the dotted line, through the named branches and the cervical dermatomes as shown.

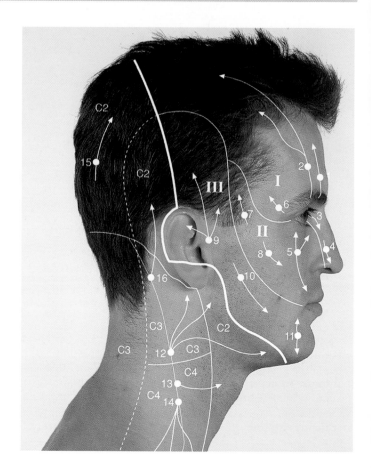

3.15
Cutaneous innervation of the head and neck

1	Supratrochlear	9	Auriculotemporal
2	Supraorbital	10	Buccal
3	Infratrochlear	11	Mental
4	External nasal	12	Greater auricular
5	Infraorbital	13	Transverse cervical
6	Lacrimal	14	Supraclavicular
7	Zygomaticotemporal	15	Greater occipital
8	Zygomaticofacial	16	Lesser occipital

I, II, III Ophthalmic, maxillary and mandibular divisions of the trigeminal nerve

LYMPH NODES OF THE HEAD AND NECK

The lymphatic drainage of the head and neck is through deep and superficial lymphatic rings, around the base of the skull, and the deep and superficial lymph chains. The deep ring around the oro- and nasopharynx includes the palatine tonsil. The superficial ring comprises the occipital, retroauricular, superficial and deep parotid, submandibular and submental nodes. The deep cervical lymph chain lies around the internal jugular vein, prominent nodes being in the carotid triangle, around the digastric and omohyoid muscles, and in the posterior triangle above the clavicle. Superficial lymph chains lie along the external and anterior jugular veins.

Enlarged cervical lymph nodes are the commonest neck lumps seen in clinical practice. They are usually associated with tonsillar or upper respiratory tract infection but may also be the site of metastases from malignancies of the nasal cavities, thyroid gland, lungs and breast. Occasionally, malignancy of the upper abdomen can present with enlargement of a left supraclavicular node.

The order of palpation of cervical lymph nodes is not critical, provided all groups are included. They may be examined from the front, or from behind as for the thyroid gland. In the former, simultaneous examination of the two sides can be undertaken with the pulps of the second, third and fourth fingers of both hands. Examined in turn are the occipital, retroauricular, superficial and deep parotid, submandibular and submental lymph nodes. This is followed by palpation downwards, along the anterior border of the sternocleidomastoid muscle to the clavicle, palpating the internal jugular lymph chain.

An enlarged node can be missed deep to the lower end of the sternocleidomastoid muscle if not carefully searched for by gently squeezing the finger and thumb deep to the lower end of the muscle. Passing backwards from this area, the supraclavicular nodes are examined and then, by ascending along the posterior border of the sternocleidomastoid muscle, the external jugular lymph chain. Additional nodes may be present anterior to the larynx and along the anterior jugular vein.

3

3.16
Lymph nodes of the head and neck
1 Mental
2 Submandibular
3 Parotid
4 Retroauricular
5 Occipital
6 Digastric
7 Omohyoid
8 Supraclavicular
9 Deep cervical lymph chain around the internal jugular vein
10 Superficial cervical lymph chains around external and anterior jugular veins

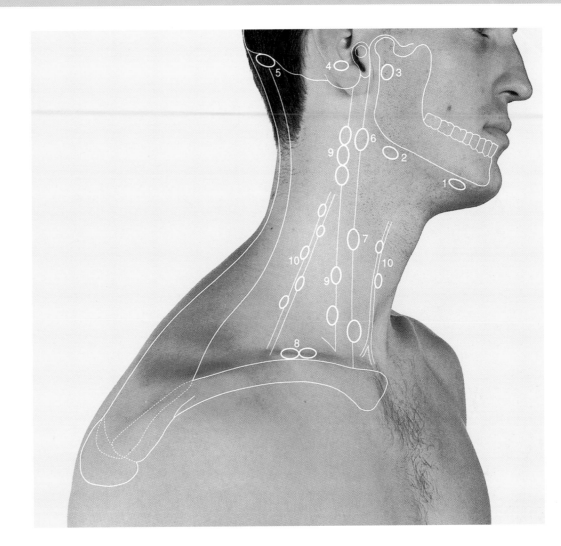

4 THORAX

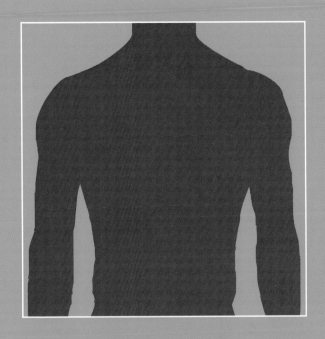

ANTERIOR CHEST WALL

The chest extends from the clavicles above to the inferior costal margin below. It is formed of the ribs and costal cartilages, the sternum and associated muscles; the two sides of the chest are usually symmetrical. The rate, depth and character of respiration can be observed, as can the apex beat of the heart on the left side. The midline sternum is made up of the manubrium, the body and the xiphisternum from above downwards (Fig. 4.2). The suprasternal notch on the superior aspect of the manubrium is palpable. The manubrium and body are also palpable throughout their length and they are united by a secondary cartilaginous joint forming the sternal angle (the angle of Louis). The angle is at the level of the lower border of the fourth thoracic vertebral body. It forms an important landmark for the description of structures inside the chest. Ribs are counted from this site, as it is consistently palpable: the second costal cartilage articulates on each side of the manubriosternal joint. The xiphisternum is covered by the rectus abdominis muscles and is less easily palpable. It is of variable length and when long, and suddenly noted by a subject, may be thought to be abnormal. The xiphisternal joint is at the level of the ninth thoracic vertebral body.

The rib cage is made up of 12 pairs of ribs, each having a posterolateral bony and an anterior costal cartilaginous component (Fig. 4.2). In a thin male subject, many ribs are visible but they may be obscured by overlying muscle, fat or breast tissue. These structures can also make it difficult to count ribs by palpation. The first rib is not easily palpated, being deep to the fibres of the pectoralis major muscle and the clavicle. The second is consistently palpable at its cartilaginous articulation with the manubriosternal junction. The upper seven (true) ribs articulate directly with the sternum via their costal cartilages, whereas the eighth to 10th (false) ribs articulate via their costal cartilages

with the cartilage of the rib above. The 11th and 12th (floating) ribs are considered in Figure 4.7. The lower costal margin is formed by the lower six ribs and their costal cartilages. The number of the ribs and intercostal spaces are used when describing normal and abnormal findings of the chest wall or thoracic cavity. The intercostal spaces are filled by the intercostal muscles, attached to the adjacent ribs.

The clavicle is palpable throughout its length; it articulates medially at the sternoclavicular joint. Like the temporomandibular joint, it has a fibrocartilaginous covering of its articular surfaces and contains a fibrocartilaginous disc. The pectoralis major muscle is attached medially to the clavicle and upper five to seven costal cartilages, their related half of the sternum, and from the sheath of the rectus abdominis (Fig. 4.5). Its fibres pass laterally to the lateral lip of the bicipital groove of the humerus and form the bulk of the anterior axillary fold (Fig. 4.12). The pectoralis minor muscle is overlapped by the pectoralis major, but its tendon may be palpable high in the anterior axillary wall as it passes to the coracoid process. The process can be felt by deep palpation 1 cm below the clavicle under the medial anterior fibres of the deltoid muscle.

The deltoid muscle forms the rounded contour of the shoulder overlapping the shoulder joint. The muscles of the abdominal wall gain a wide attachment to the lower ribs and costal cartilages and are considered in Figure 5.2.

Severe injury to the chest wall can fracture the ribs. Although this is a painful condition, bony union is usually uncomplicated. However, the fractured bone ends may damage the underlying lung, producing leakage of air into the pleural cavity (pneumothorax), or lacerate other adjacent viscera, notably the liver and spleen.

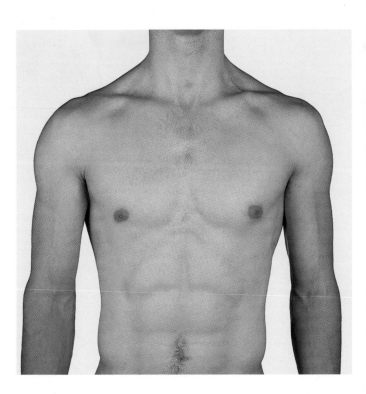

4.1
Anterior chest wall

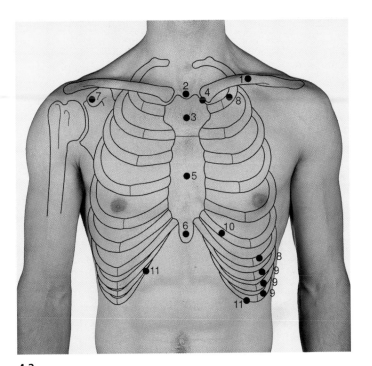

4.2
Anterior chest wall: bones

1 Clavicle	7 Coracoid process
2 Suprasternal notch	8 True ribs
3 Manubrium	9 False ribs
4 Sternoclavicular joint	10 Costal cartilages
5 Body of sternum	11 Costal margin
6 Xiphisternum	

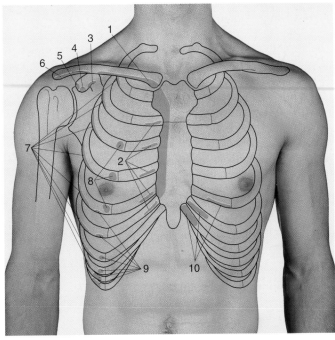

4.4
Anterior chest wall: muscle attachments

1 and 2 Pectoralis major	6 Deltoid
3 and 8 Pectoralis minor	7 Serratus anterior
4 Coracobrachialis	9 External oblique
5 Short head of biceps	10 Rectus abdominis

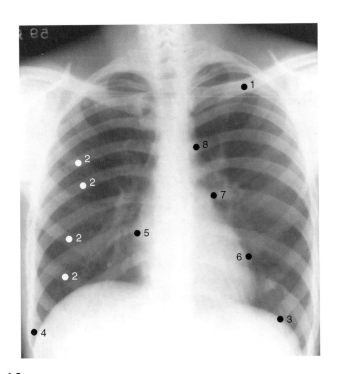

4.3
Chest radiograph: anterior view

1 Clavicle	5 Right border of heart
2 Ribs	6 Left border of heart
3 Left dome of diaphragm	7 Pulmonary conus
4 Right costophrenic angle	8 Aortic knuckle

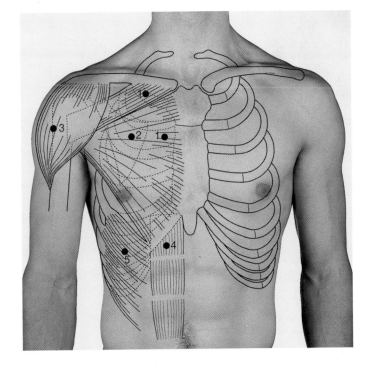

4.5
Anterior chest wall: muscles

1 Pectoralis major	4 Rectus abdominis
2 Pectoralis minor	5 External oblique
3 Deltoid	

ANTERIOR THORAX, PLEURA AND LUNGS

The lower three cervical, and all the thoracic, vertebral spines are palpable in the midline. The spine and acromion of the scapula are subcutaneous and its upper, lower and medial angles can be observed and palpated during arm movements. In the anatomical position, the scapula overlies the second to seventh ribs on the posterolateral aspect of the chest wall. Laterally it articulates with the clavicle and humerus but has no medial bony attachment, being free to move over the chest wall in movements of the upper limb (Fig. 7.14, p. 69). Much of the rib cage is impalpable posteriorly, being covered by powerful erector spinae muscles alongside the midline and the scapula and its muscle attachments more laterally. The 11th and 12th (floating) ribs articulate with their respective vertebrae but are free laterally and these ends can be palpated and this mobility confirmed.

Pleura and lungs (Figs 4.6, 4.7)

Each pleural cavity extends superiorly 3 cm above the middle of the medial third of the clavicle and the possibility of damage in surgical procedures in the neck is considered in Figure 3.14 (p. 27). The anterior border of the pleural cavity reaches the midline at the sternal angle. The left moves away from the midline at the fourth costal cartilage, the right at the sixth costal cartilage and both cross the midclavicular line at the eighth costal cartilage, the midaxillary line at the 10th cartilage and pass along the line of the 12th rib posteriorly (to be remembered by the even numbers). These markings indicate the extent of the pleura around the outer chest wall. The diaphragm bulges up into each pleural cavity from below, reaching as high as the fourth intercostal space on the right side and the fifth on the left. The cardiac notch on the left side, at the fourth costal cartilage, is produced by the heart which bulges into the medial surface of both cavities but more markedly on the left.

The lung markings coincide with those of the pleura, except inferiorly, where they do not extend down into the lateral recesses and are approximately two rib spaces higher. The oblique fissure of each lung, separating its upper and lower lobes, follows a line from the third thoracic vertebra to the sixth costochondral junction. The horizontal fissure, dividing the right upper and middle lobes, follows a horizontal line from the oblique fissure to the fourth right costal cartilage. The position of the trachea in the neck is always identified when examining the lungs and pleural cavities. It should lie in the midline deep to the sternal notch and a finger will pass into the slight hollow on either side of it. The trachea divides at the level of the sternal angle.

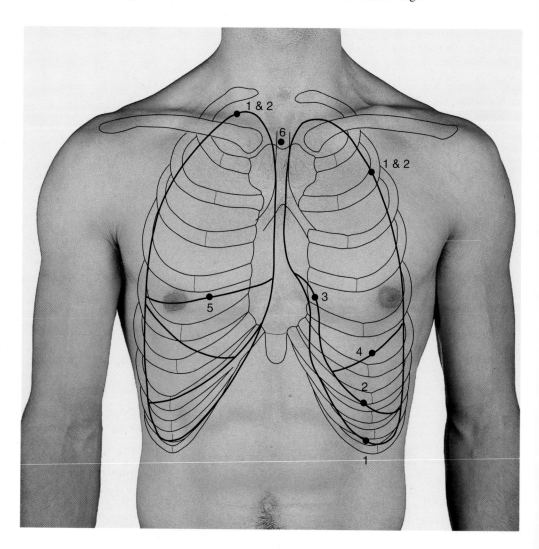

4.6
Surface markings of the lungs and pleura
1 Pleural markings
2 Lung markings
3 Cardiac notch
4 Oblique fissure
5 Horizontal fissure
6 Trachea

POSTERIOR THORAX, PLEURA AND LUNGS

Respiratory movements can be magnified by placing the flat of each hand on the chest wall with the thumbs pointing towards each other near the midline. The hands are separated and the ribs are more horizontally placed in inspiration than in expiration. Reverberation felt with the flat of the hand over the chest wall when a subject talks is known as tactile vocal fremitus. This is accentuated in certain lung diseases. The lungs are resonant to percussion, as can be demonstrated over the clavicles, the upper chest and the axillary regions. When percussing from the left axilla towards the midline, a duller sound is heard and felt as the left border of the heart is encountered. The right border of the heart usually lies near the sternum and is not easily detected in the normal person. It is generally easier to detect borders by percussion from resonant to dull. Percussion downwards from the clavicle on the right side will demonstrate the dull sound produced by the upper border of the liver at about the fourth intercostal space.

If the bell of a stethoscope is pressed onto the upper chest in the midaxillary line, air will be heard to enter the lungs in inspiration, the noise extending slightly into the beginning of expiration. The sound stops during the remainder of expiration.

This normal pattern is known as vesicular breathing. If the stethoscope is placed over the larynx, noise will be heard during both inspiration and expiration with a break in-between. This is known as bronchial breathing. The latter pattern may also occur over the peripheral area of the chest in certain lung diseases. If the patient speaks during auscultation the sound is transmitted to the chest wall; this is known as vocal resonance and its character may be altered by lung disease. In disease there may also be added noise to the respiratory pattern. Inflammation of the lung (pneumonia) fills the alveoli with purulent exudate, reducing oxygen transfer and producing dyspnoea (breathlessness). The breath sounds in the consolidated lung become more prominent. The sounds are reduced if a part of the lung collapses (atelectasis), or when fluid (effusion) or air (pneumothorax) collects in the pleural cavity.

The trapezius and latissimus dorsi muscles have attachments to the trunk. Their prime function is in movement of the shoulder girdle; they are considered in Figure 7.14 (p. 69). The deltoid muscle forms the rounded contour of the shoulder, gaining attachment from the clavicle and the scapula (Fig. 7.9, p. 67).

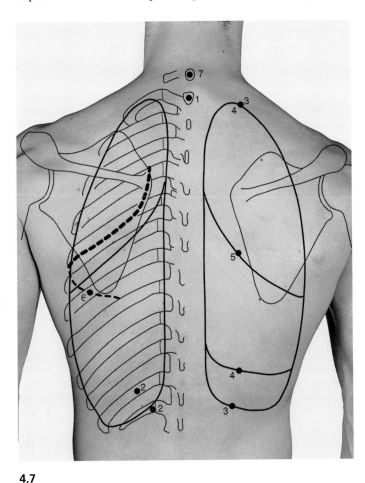

4.7
Posterior chest wall: ribs, lungs and pleura
1 Spine of first thoracic vertebra
2 Floating ribs
3 Pleural markings
4 Lung markings
5 Oblique fissure
6 Posterolateral thoracotomy incision
7 Vertebra prominens

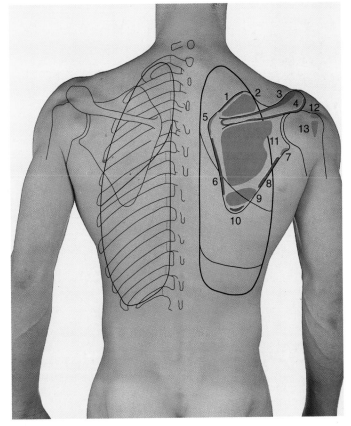

4.8
Posterior chest wall: muscle attachments
1 Levator scapulae
2 and 12 Supraspinatus
3 Trapezius
4 Deltoid
5 Rhomboideus major
6 Rhomboideus minor
7 Long head of triceps
8 and 13 Teres minor
9 Teres major
10 Latissimus dorsi
11 and 12 Infraspinatus

ANTERIOR THORAX, HEART AND GREAT VESSELS

The thoracic cavity can be divided into a central (mediastinal) region and, on each side, a pleural cavity containing a lung. The mediastinum is divided for descriptive purposes into superior, above a horizontal plane joining the sternal angle to the lower part of the body of the fourth thoracic vertebra, and, below this line, into a central part containing the heart and the anterior and posterior mediastinum, in front of and behind the heart. The apex of the heart is usually in the left midclavicular line in the fifth intercostal space (Fig. 4.9). The inferior ('acute') border passes horizontally from this point across the midline and the right border bulges slightly laterally along the right border of the sternum. The left ('obtuse') border curves from the apex upwards and medially to the sternal end of the second left inter-costal space. Figure 4.9 indicates the cardiac chambers, sulci and great vessel roots that constitute these borders. The surface markings of the valves indicate the atrioventricular junction and the origin of the aorta and pulmonary trunk (Fig. 4.10). The aortic arch, curving posteriorly and to the left, is sited in the superior mediastinum.

The innominate artery bifurcation lies behind the right sterno-clavicular joint and the subclavian arteries arch over the apex of each lung (Fig. 4.11). The brachiocephalic veins are formed by the union of the internal jugular and subclavian veins, just lateral to the sternoclavicular joint. The right vein descends vertically along the right border of the sternum and the left crosses obliquely behind the manubrium; they join at the level of the sternal angle to form the superior vena cava. The inferior vena caval opening through the diaphragm is just to the right of the xiphisternum at the level of the eighth thoracic vertebra. The descending thoracic aorta and the oesophagus are sited in the posterior mediastinum and pass through the diaphragm at the level of the 12th and 10th thoracic vertebrae, respectively. These marked differences in vertebral levels (eighth, 10th and 12th) reflect the steep half-domed nature of the diaphragm (high ante-riorly and low posteriorly) and the relative anteroposterior posi-tions of the orifices. The apex beat of the heart can usually be felt by placing the flat of the hand over the left side of the chest, centred over the fifth intercostal space in the midclavicular line.

On listening over the heart, two distinct noises are heard close together at the beginning of each beat. These are usually referred to as 'lubb-dupp'. The first is produced by the closure of the mitral and tricuspid valves and the second by the aortic and pul-monary valves. Each valve is heard most clearly over specific areas of the anterior chest. The two valves in the systemic circu-lation provide most of the noise. The mitral valve is heard best over the apex of the heart. If this is not palpable, the stethoscope

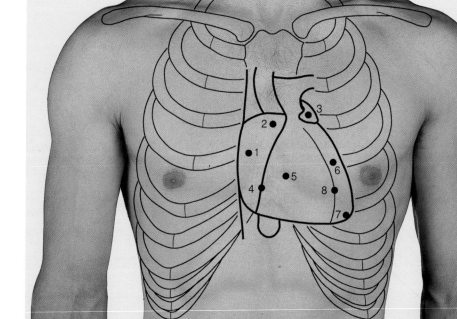

4.9
Surface markings of the chambers of the heart
1 Right atrium
2 Right auricular appendage
3 Left auricular appendage
4 Coronary sulcus
5 Right ventricle
6 Left ventricle
7 Apex of heart
8 Anterior interventricular sulcus

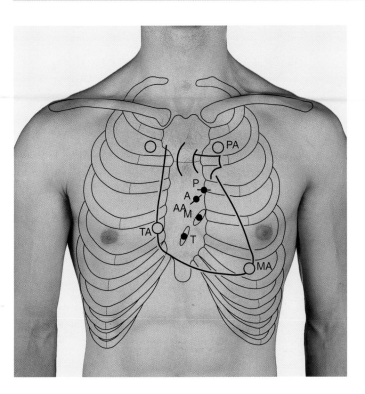

4.10
Surface markings of the cardiac valves and their optimal sites for auscultation (A)

T Tricuspid	M Mitral
P Pulmonary	A Aortic

4.11
Surface markings of the great vessels of the superior mediastinum

1 Aortic arch	5 Right brachiocephalic vein
2 Innominate (brachiocephalic) artery	6 Left brachiocephalic vein
3 Left common carotid artery	7 Superior vena cava
4 Left subclavian artery	8 Inferior vena cava

should be placed over the left fifth intercostal space in line with the nipple (the midclavicular line). Auscultation of this area in the female may require raising a pendulous breast. The aortic area is just to the right of the sternum in the first intercostal space and the pulmonary area at an equivalent site to the left of the sternum. The tricuspid area is over the right side of the sternum at the level of the fourth costal cartilage. Abnormalities of the heart and valves may alter or produce additional hearts sounds.

Disease of the coronary arteries compromises the blood supplied to the heart muscle. This may produce pain on exercise, i.e. when the muscle requires more blood, a condition known as angina. Severe deprivation of the blood supply to the myocardium may produce an area of cardiac muscle death (myocardial infarction, MI). Infarction interferes with muscle contraction and may also damage the conducting system of the heart, giving rise to abnormal rhythms, possibly with a fatal result.

LATERAL CHEST WALL, BREAST AND AXILLA

The lateral chest wall is bounded inferiorly by the lower edge of the rib cage and superiorly it projects into the axilla. It is continuous with the anterior and posterior chest wall without any demarcating line (Fig. 4.12). Ribs can usually be palpated along the length of this wall but, as the topmost rib felt in the axilla varies, counting is either from the floating ribs or by following a numbered rib from the sternum. The serratus anterior muscle is attached along the length of the anterior medial border of the scapula; its fibres pass laterally and form eight slips, attached to the upper eight ribs. These slips can be seen in a thin subject, together with their interdigitations with the external oblique muscle on the middle four ribs. It is supplied by the long thoracic nerve, from the brachial plexus.

The female breast extends from the second to the seventh ribs and from the lateral border of the sternum to the anterior axillary wall. It overlies the pectoralis major, the serratus anterior and the external oblique muscles (Fig. 4.14). The axillary tail of the breast extends superolaterally around the lower border of the pectoralis major muscle into the axilla. The size of the breast and level of the nipple are variable in the female. In the male the nipple is in the midclavicular line over the fourth intercostal space.

4

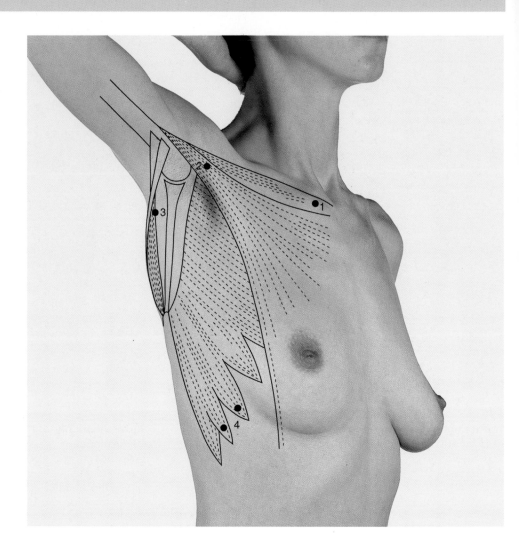

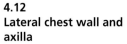

4.12
Lateral chest wall and axilla
1 Clavicle
2 Anterior axillary fold
3 Posterior axillary fold
4 Slips of the serratus anterior passing onto lateral aspect of ribs

The axilla is a fat-filled pyramidal cavity separating the chest and arm. Its medial wall is formed by the upper six ribs and the anterior and posterior walls converge laterally onto the palpable upper shaft of the humerus. The anterior and posterior walls can be felt between finger and thumb; the anterior is higher and is formed mainly of the pectoralis major muscle (Fig. 4.14). The posterior wall is mainly from the teres major muscle, passing from the medial edge of the scapula to the medial lip of the bicipital groove of the humerus; the tendon of latissimus dorsi wraps around the inferior border of the teres major muscle. The apex of the axilla leads into the neck through a narrow opening, the cervico-axillary canal. This transmits the axillary vessels and the cords of the brachial plexus. The artery can be palpated laterally on the posterior axillary wall. The cords of the brachial plexus are closely applied to the axillary artery within the axillary sheath; local anaesthetic can be injected into the sheath to spread along it to produce regional anaesthesia. The axilla contains many lymph nodes and is covered inferiorly by skin arching from the chest wall onto the arm.

The breast is palpated for abnormal masses with the flat of the hand, compressing it against the chest wall. Its mobility over underlying muscle is assessed by subjects pressing their hands on their hips. Malignancy of the breast may spread to lymph nodes in the axilla. These nodes may also be involved in infection and malignancy at other sites. The nodes are sited in anterior, posterior, medial, lateral and apical groups; the apical group is high in the axilla, communicating through the cervico-axillary canal with the supraclavicular nodes and lymph channels forming the subclavian lymph trunk (Fig. 4.15). Normal axillary lymph nodes may be palpable, mainly as small nodules of 4–8 mm in diameter, often termed 'shotty' nodes.

The axillary contents are palpated with the subject's arm slightly abducted, flexed at the elbow and with the hand resting on the chest. The examiner's left hand is used to examine the right axilla and the right hand the left axilla. During this manoeuvre, the non-palpating hand holds the elbow of the subject to support the weight of the arm. The apical and medial nodes are palpated with a cupped hand passing up the lateral aspect of the axilla, feeling the axillary contents against the chest wall as the hand is drawn downwards. Other groups of lymph nodes are examined by compressing the axillary contents against the anterior and posterior axillary walls and laterally against the humerus.

THORACIC INCISIONS AND ACCESS POINTS

The majority of cardiac operations are undertaken through a midline sternal splitting incision. After dividing the skin and subcutaneous tissues the bone is divided by a vibrating bone saw or specific bone-cutting instruments. On separating the two halves of the sternum the chest wall and pleural cavities are pulled laterally exposing the pericardium and great vessels. The left brachiocephalic vein crosses the superior mediastinum and is put on a stretch by this manoeuvre; it has to be carefully freed to avoid damage.

The ventricles, mitral valve and pulmonary trunk may also be exposed through an incision following the anterolateral aspect of the left fifth rib. The incision passes through skin and subcutaneous tissue onto the rib and the periosteum is divided along the outside of the rib. By stripping the periosteum from the inferior margin of the rib a further incision can be made through the periosteum and parietal pleura in the rib bed to enter the pleural cavity. In this incision the rib is not removed but may be divided posteriorly, or the incision taken transversely across the sternum, to obtain greater exposure.

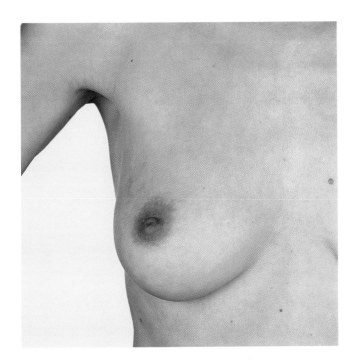

4.13
Female breast

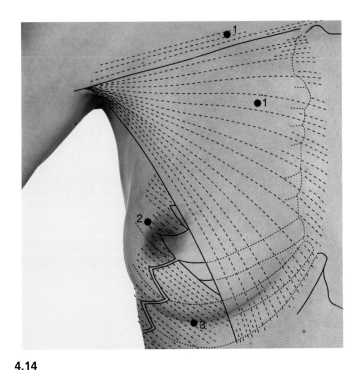

4.14
Female breast: relation to the chest wall
1 Pectoralis major   3 External oblique
2 Serratus anterior

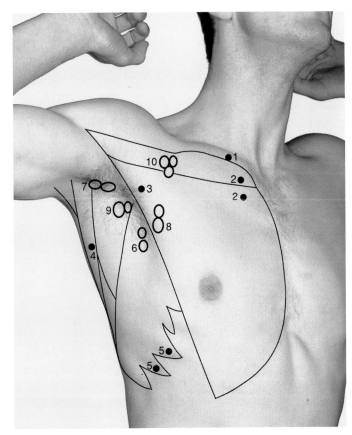

4.15
Axillary lymph nodes
1 Clavicle
2 Pectoralis major
3 Anterior axillary fold
4 Tendon of latissimus dorsi
5 Serratus anterior

6–10 Groups of nodes:
 6 Medial
 7 Lateral
 8 Anterior
 9 Posterior
10 Apical

To expose the hilum of the lung, a posterolateral incision is made through the chest wall with the patient lying on the opposite side and the free arm flexed to pull the scapula forward around the rib cage. The incision follows the line of the fourth rib and fibres of the trapezius and latissimus dorsi muscles are divided in line with the incision. Exposure of the posterior mediastinum is through the bed of the seventh or eighth ribs. This incision may be continued across the costal margin to open the abdominal cavity as in operations on the gastro-oesophageal junction.

An intracardiac injection can be made through the medial aspect of the fifth intercostal space. A needle inserted alongside the xiphisternum and passed cranially deep to the body of the sternum will enter the pericardial cavity.

The intercostal nerves run deep to the inferior margin of each rib and they can be anaesthetised by injection of local anaesthetic for pain relief. The site chosen is usually along the posterior axillary line deep to the inferior border of one or more ribs.

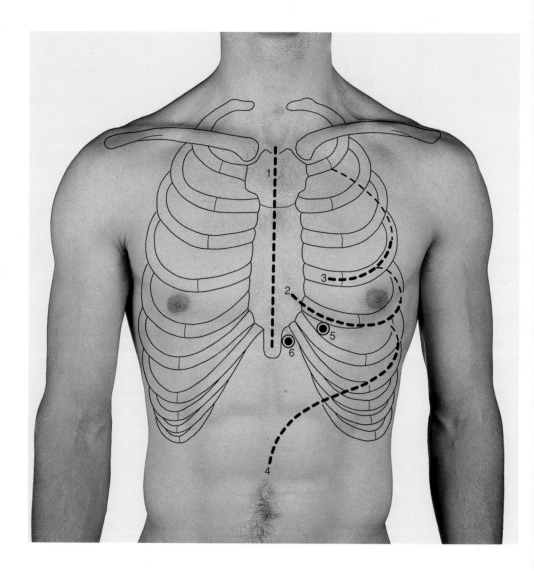

4.16
Applied anatomy of the anterior chest wall
1 Midline sternotomy approach to the mediastinum
2 Left anterolateral thoracotomy through bed of fifth rib
3 Posterolateral thoracotomy through bed of fourth rib
4 Thoraco-abdominal incision
5 Point for insertion of a needle into ventricles
6 Point for insertion of a needle into pericardial cavity

5 ABDOMEN AND PELVIS

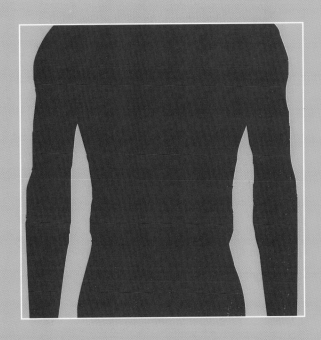

ANTERIOR ABDOMINAL WALL

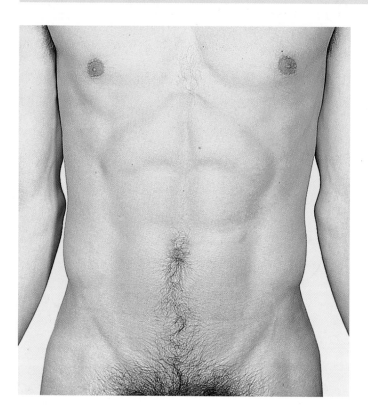

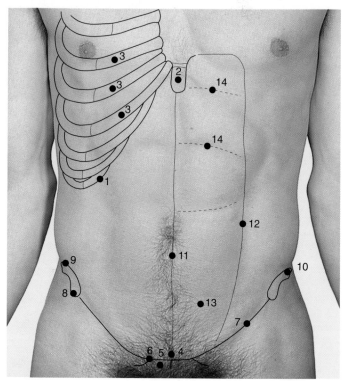

5.1
Anterior abdominal wall

5.2
Anterior abdominal wall: bones

1 Costal margin	8 Anterior superior iliac
2 Xiphisternum	spine
3 Fifth, sixth and seventh	9 Iliac crest
costal cartilages	10 Iliac tubercle
4 Symphysis pubis	11 Linea alba
5 Body of pubis	12 Linea semilunaris
6 Pubic tubercle	13 Rectus abdominis muscle
7 Inguinal ligament	14 Tendinous intersections

The anterior abdominal wall is bounded superiorly by the lower costal margin and inferiorly by the symphysis pubis, the pubic crest and tubercle, the inguinal ligament, the anterior superior iliac spine and the iliac crest, from medial to lateral (Fig. 5.2). The wall comprises three flat sheet-like muscles. They fuse medially to form a fibrous sheath for the vertically running rectus abdominis muscles, lying on each side of the midline. The sheaths of the two sides meet in the midline as a fibrous raphe, known as the linea alba. The three transverse lines of attachment of the rectus abdominis muscle to the anterior sheath can be seen in a muscular subject above the umbilicus; they are termed tendinous intersections. The superior end of the rectus abdominis muscle crosses the anterior rib cage to be attached to the fifth, sixth and seventh costal cartilages from lateral to medial. The lateral line of formation of the rectus sheath is known as the linea semilunaris.

The most superficial of the three sheet-like abdominal muscles is the external oblique; it is attached superiorly by slips to the lateral aspect of the lower eight ribs and interdigitates with the serratus anterior over the middle four ribs. Medially, the muscle forms part of the rectus sheath and interiorly it is attached to the symphysis pubis, pubic tubercle, anterior superior iliac spine and the anterior half of the iliac crest. The muscle is extensively aponeurotic (visible in Fig. 5.1) medial to, and below, a line skirting the costal attachments of rectus abdominis, descending vertically from the ninth costal cartilage to below

the umbilicus. It then curves laterally towards the anterior superior iliac spine. Between the spine and the pubic tubercle, the aponeurotic edge is recurved on itself to form the inguinal ligament. The muscle has a free posterior border but this is not usually visible or palpable in a living subject. The muscles of the anterior abdominal wall are supplied by the lower five intercostal, the subcostal and the first lumbar nerves.

The anterior abdominal wall is divided for descriptive purposes into nine regions by two horizontal lines (subcostal and transtubercular) and two vertical lines through the midpoint of each clavicle (Fig. 5.4 – these lines cross the costal margin at the tip of the ninth costal cartilage and the midinguinal point; see p. 48). The subcostal plane passes through the lower border of the third lumbar vertebra; the transtubercular plane passes through the iliac tubercle and the fifth lumbar spine. The three central regions formed by these lines are the epigastrium, umbilical and suprapubic, from above downwards. The three regions on each side are the hypochondrium, lumbar and iliac, from

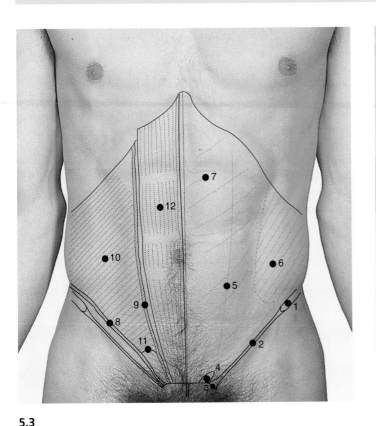

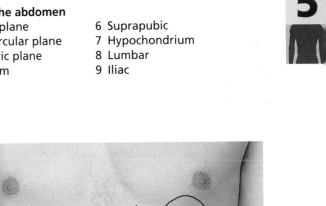

5.3
Anterior abdominal wall: muscles

1 Anterior superior iliac spine	7 Tendinous intersections of rectus abdominis
2 Inguinal ligament	8,9 Cut edges of external oblique
3 Pubic tubercle	
4 Superficial inguinal ring	10 Internal oblique muscle fibres
5 External oblique aponeurosis	11 Conjoint tendon
6 External oblique muscle fibres	12 Rectus abdominis muscle

5.4
Regions of the abdomen

1 Subcostal plane	6 Suprapubic
2 Transtubercular plane	7 Hypochondrium
3 Transpyloric plane	8 Lumbar
4 Epigastrium	9 Iliac
5 Umbilical	

5

above downwards. Another plane sometimes referred to in clinical practice is the horizontal, transduodenal (transpyloric) plane, passing through the first part of the duodenum. It is at the level of the lower border of the first lumbar vertebra; ventrally, the transpyloric plane lies midway between the xiphisternal joint and the umbilicus. The abdominal cavity extends upwards behind the lower ribs and downwards into the pelvis.

Surface markings of the alimentary tract (Fig. 5.5)
The oesophagus passes through the diaphragm at the level of the 10th thoracic vertebra, just to the left of the midline. The duodenum starts variably to the right of the midline, sometimes in,

5.5
Surface markings of the alimentary tract

1 Oesophagus	8 Appendix (in pelvic position)
2 Stomach	
3 Pyloric antrum	9 Ascending colon
4 Duodenum	10 Transverse colon
5 Duodenojejunal flexure	11 Descending colon
6 Terminal ileum	12 Sigmoid colon
7 Caecum	

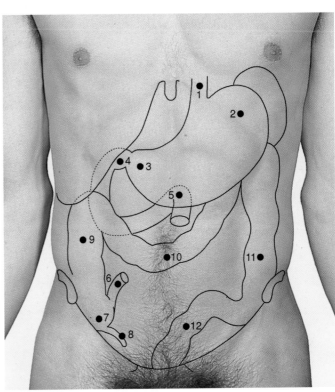

5

but frequently far below, the transpyloric plane. The stomach lies between these two points and is of variable size, partly covered by the rib cage and filling the epigastrium. The duodenum curves in C fashion, convex to the right, to end at the duodenojejunal flexure, this being sited near the midline and approximately in the subcostal plane. The root of the small gut mesentery passes obliquely over the posterior abdominal wall from the flexure to the right iliac fossa, and the central abdomen and upper pelvis are filled with loops of small gut.

The base of the appendix is sited in the right iliac fossa, the surface marking being approximately at the junction of the middle and lateral thirds of a line joining the umbilicus to the anterior superior iliac spine. Initially, inflammation of the appendix produces referred pain around the umbilicus (i.e. the 10th thoracic dermatome) but, as it progresses and involves the parietal peritoneum, local tenderness becomes more marked in the right iliac fossa. The tip of the appendix is usually positioned laterally, inferior to, or behind the caecum, but it may pass downwards into the pelvis or be related to the terminal ileum. The caecum, ascending colon and hepatic flexure of the colon on the

right side, and the splenic flexure descending colon on the left, are largely retroperitoneal structures whereas the transverse and sigmoid colons have a mesentery and vary in their position, although they are usually in the regions shown (Fig. 5.5).

Pain produced by inflammation of part of the gut may initially be referred, e.g. the small gut and appendix to the umbilical region, and the large gut to the suprapubic region. However, once the inflammation affects the adjacent parietal peritoneum, the pain and associated tenderness become focal to the area of disease.

Surface markings of non-alimentary tract viscera (Figs. 5.7, 5.10)

The liver lies in the right hypochondrium above the costal margin. Its upper border, bulging into the diaphragm, is at the level of the fourth intercostal space. The left lobe passes deep to the xiphisternum across the epigastrium. The gall bladder projects just below the liver at the point where the midclavicular line crosses the costal margin, i.e. the ninth costal cartilage. The spleen is situated posteriorly along the line of the left ninth to 11th ribs. The kidneys lie on the posterior abdominal wall (Fig. 5.10). The pancreas passes from the concavity of the duodenum, slightly obliquely upwards across the midline, over the posterior abdominal wall; its tail passes into the hilum of the spleen.

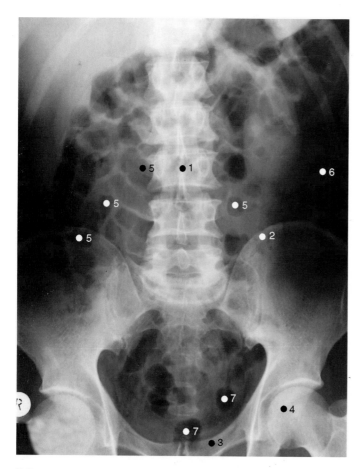

5.6
Abdomen: plain abdominal radiograph

1 Third lumbar vertebra
2 Ilium
3 Superior ramus of pubis
4 Head of femur
5 Gas shadows in small gut
6 Gas shadows in left colon
7 Gas shadows in rectum

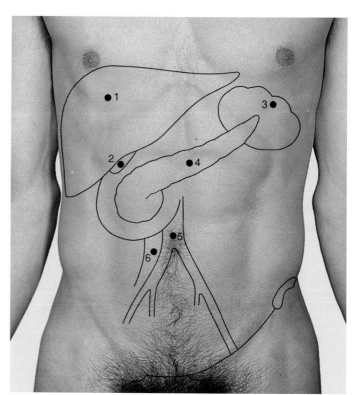

5.7
Surface marking of non-alimentary tract abdominal viscera
(The structures labelled 3–6 lie on the posterior abdominal wall)

1 Liver
2 Gall bladder
3 Spleen
4 Pancreas
5 Aortic bifurcation
6 Formation of inferior vena cava

The abdominal aorta lies on the posterior abdominal wall near the midline and to the left of the inferior vena cava. It divides at the level of the umbilicus, at the level of the body of the fourth lumbar vertebra. The common and external iliac arteries pass from the umbilicus to the midinguinal point (midway between the anterior superior iliac spine and the symphysis pubis) to continue as the femoral artery. The inferior vena cava is formed at the level of the body of the fifth lumbar vertebra, its common iliac tributaries lying to the right and posterior to their respective arteries. The external iliac and femoral veins lie medial to their respective arteries. Note that the umbilicus varies at the level of the disc between the third and fourth lumbar vertebrae in young muscular adults, but descends over the body of the fourth lumbar vertebra in middle age.

ABDOMINAL INCISIONS

Most abdominal viscera can be reached through a midline incision (Fig. 5.8). This may be in the upper or lower abdomen, or along its full length, depending on the target organ. The incision divides the skin, the two layers of superficial fascia and the fibres of the linea alba, this being wide enough to divide in the midline without entering either rectus sheath. The transversalis fascia and peritoneum are also divided in the line of the skin incision.

The liver and gall bladder may be conveniently approached through a right subcostal incision. The rectus muscle and anterior and posterior rectus sheath are divided in line with the incision, as are the three sheath-like abdominal muscles. A left subcostal incision can be used to approach the spleen and the left and right subcostal incisions can be combined across the midline (rooftop incision) to give a wide bilateral access to the kidneys and suprarenal glands.

The bladder, and the uterus and its adnexia, can be approached through a transverse suprapubic (Pfannenstiel) incision. The skin, two layers of superficial fascia and the anterior rectus sheath are divided in line with the incision. The rectus abdominis muscles are not adherent to the sheath at this level and can be retracted laterally to expose the transversalis fascia and peritoneum; these structures are divided in line with the skin incision. It is possible to approach the inferior aspect of the bladder and the prostate gland in a plane posterior to the symphysis pubis using the suprapubic approach, retracting the peritoneum but not dividing it, i.e. staying outside the peritoneal cavity.

The appendix is approached through an oblique incision about 3 cm above and medial to the anterior superior iliac spine, dividing the skin and two layers of superficial fascia. The external oblique muscle fibres run in the same plane and are separated in this line. The internal oblique and transverse abdominus muscles, running in a different plane, are also split in line with their fibres from the centre of the incision so that, when repaired at the end of the procedure, the lines of division overlap each other in a gridiron fashion. A wider approach to the appendix can be obtained by dividing the three abdominal wall muscles in line with a longer oblique skin incision, and a similar left iliac incision can be used to approach the sigmoid colon.

A transverse incision through the rectus muscle in the transpyloric plane is used to approach the gastroduodenal junction in babies with abnormalities of this region. Although the kidney can be reached from anteriorly, its posterior position favours a more posterior approach. A wide exposure can be obtained through an incision along the line of the 12th rib, the abdominal wall muscles being divided and the kidney approached retroperitoneally (Fig. 5.10).

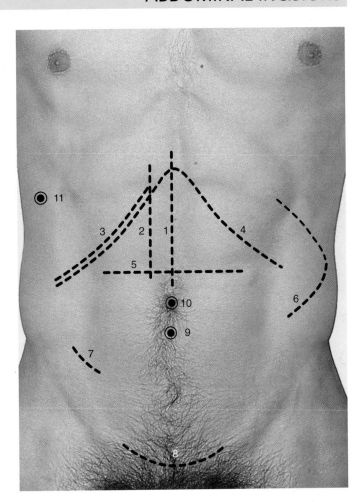

5.8
Abdominal incisions: anterior
1 Midline
2 Paramedian
3 Subcostal
4 Roof top
5 Transverse
6 Renal
7 Appendix
8 Suprapubic
9 Point for insertion of peritoneal catheter
10 Point for insertion of laparoscope
11 Access point for liver biopsy

A needle may be inserted into the liver usually through the right seventh intercostal space in the anterior axillary line. The needle passes through the lateral recess of the pleural cavity and the diaphragm but does not pass through the lung; the needle is inserted with the subject holding a breath in expiration. The procedure may be used to obtain a liver biopsy or to introduce radio-opaque material into an obstructed dilated biliary system.

Other commonly undertaken biopsies are of the kidney, through the site of its posterior surface marking.

A needle may be passed into the peritoneal cavity, in a site such as the iliac fossa, to identify and sample any abnormal peritoneal fluid. Peritoneal tubes for renal dialysis can be inserted through the linea alba 2 cm below the umbilicus; the dialysate is introduced and then syphoned off after a number of hours.

POSTERIOR ABDOMINAL WALL

In the posterior lower trunk, the lower ribs, iliac crest, posterior superior and inferior iliac spines, lumbar spines and the posterior aspect of the sacrum are palpable (Fig. 5.10). The intercristal line, joining the iliac crests, passes between the spines of the third and fourth lumbar vertebrae; often it crosses the fourth spine. Compare this with Figure 4.7 (p. 35) to relate the position of the abdominal viscera to the lungs.

The latissimus dorsi (Fig. 7.13, p. 69) takes its origin over this region and deep to it are the powerful erector spinae muscles. The spleen lies posterolateral on the left chest, deep to the ninth to 11th ribs; it is susceptible to damage by trauma of this region. The kidneys lie approximately in the transpyloric plane, the right being slightly superior. Their long axes are slightly angled, the inferior pole away from the vertical plane; they may be needled through these sites to obtain a tissue biopsy or drain an obstructed renal pelvis.

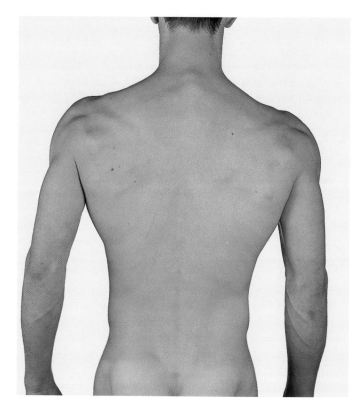

5.9
Posterior abdominal wall

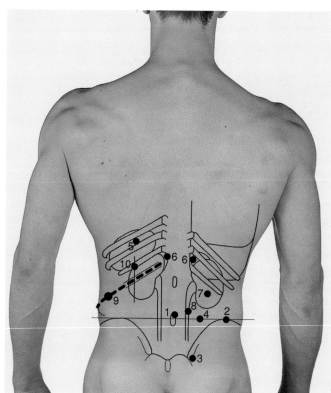

5.10
Posterior abdominal wall: bones and soft tissues

1 Fourth lumbar spine	7 Right kidney
2 Iliac crest	8 Ureters
3 Posterior superior iliac spine	9 Nephrectomy incision
4 Intercristal plane	10 Lumbotomy incision (this provides a limited exposure to the kidney and suprarenal gland)
5 Spleen	
6 Suprarenal glands	

A needle can be introduced into the aorta for the injection of radio-opaque material, demonstrating the aorta and its lower limb branches. The point of insertion is at the level of the first lumbar vertebra, 7 cm from the midline and angled 45° medially; when the needle hits the vertebral column it is gradually angled clear of the bone and then advanced forward into the aorta.

CUTANEOUS INNERVATION OF THE TRUNK

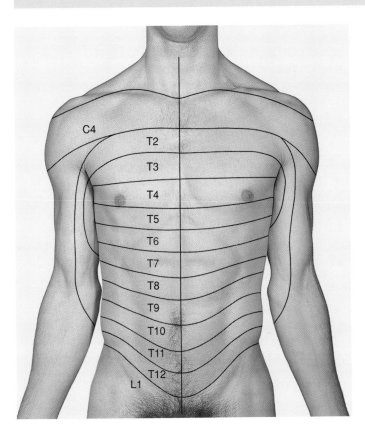

5.11
Cutaneous innervation of the trunk: anterior
The numbers denote the cutaneous innervation from the anterior primary rami of the cervical, thoracic and lumbar nerves. There is extensive overlap of consecutive dermatomes both anteriorly and posteriorly.

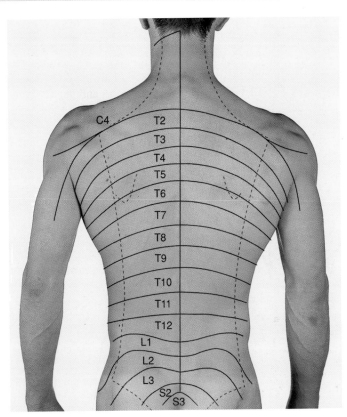

5.12
Cutaneous innervation of the trunk: posterior
The numbers denote the cutaneous innervation from the cervical, thoracic, lumbar and sacral nerves. The dotted lines enclose the areas innervated by the posterior primary rami.

ABDOMINAL EXAMINATION

The abdomen is examined with the subject lying flat on his/her back on a couch with a single pillow supporting the head and with the legs extended and uncrossed. This is the recumbent (supine) position. The abdomen is fully exposed, the breasts being covered in the female and the pubic region in both sexes until specific examination of these areas is required. The size, shape and symmetry of the abdomen are noted and the position and form of the umbilicus. At rest, respiratory movement is predominantly diaphragmatic and the abdominal wall reflects this activity. The abdominal muscles tense during coughing and on raising the head off the couch. In a thin person, central aortic pulsation and occasionally gut peristalsis may be visible. These movements are best observed by kneeling so that the examiner's eyes are at the level of the anterior abdominal wall. Not uncommonly, abnormalities such as scars of previous operations and inguinal hernias, which are protrusions of abdominal viscera through the superficial inguinal ring, may be observed. The latter are accentuated by coughing, this being referred to as an expansile cough impulse.

Palpation should be with clean, warm hands, with the observer standing on the right of the subject and the right hand carrying out most of the manoeuvres, even in a left-handed person. The hand first gently rests on the four corner regions of the abdomen in a circular order; this gentle palpation assesses muscle tone in the abdominal wall and any differences between areas. A tense abdominal wall can be felt by asking the subject to cough or raise his/her head off the pillow. In normal subjects examination produces no pain but abdominal disease may be accompanied by tenderness and this will produce protective voluntary tensing (guarding) or involuntary muscle tension (rigidity) of the abdominal wall.

Following this initial assessment of abdominal tone, each region is examined in turn, palpating for abdominal viscera and abdominal masses. It is customary to start with the right hypochondrium and then to proceed in an orderly fashion so that no region is omitted. A possible scheme is to pass on to the epi-gastrium, followed by the left hypochondrium, umbilical, left iliac, suprapubic and right iliac regions, leaving the lumbar regions until last, as these require bimanual examination. This order is sometimes related to local findings, any tender area being best left until last, but all regions must always be palpated. Palpation of posterior abdominal wall viscera and masses is by gentle depression of the relaxed anterior abdominal wall, com-pressing viscera onto the vertebral bodies and muscles of the posterior abdominal wall. The shape of any palpable organ is defined by gentle finger palpation around the area.

In the right hypochondrium, the liver edge may just be palpa-ble in a thin individual. The liver descends on inspiration and this fact is made use of for identification. The flat of the right hand is placed across the right side of the abdomen with the index finger parallel to the costal margin. The right hand is depressed into the abdomen during expiration and pressure is maintained during inspiration. The distending abdomen lifts the hand but any descending firm liver edge will be felt by the lateral border of the index finger. In enormous enlargement, the liver can extend to the right iliac fossa, so the hand is depressed first in this area and then ascends one to three fingers' breadth at a time with each res-piratory cycle, repeating the same manoeuvre until the costal margin is reached, or the edge is located.

An enlarged gall bladder moves with the liver and in line with the tip of the ninth costal cartilage, i.e. where the midclavicular line crosses the costal margin. The epigastrium contains much of the stomach, which is not usually palpable, and the left lobe of the liver which, if enlarged, is located as described above. In a thin person, the pulsation of the aorta may be felt through the stomach and pancreas. The left hypochondrium contains the rest of the stomach and the spleen may enlarge into this area. Initially splenic enlargement is below the costal margin in the left anterior axillary line but a very large spleen crosses the umbilical region and reaches the right iliac fossa. The mode of examination for the notch on the anterior edge of the spleen is the same as that for the liver, working cranially along this line of enlargement.

The semisolid contents of the colon mean that it is often pal-pable in the normal subject. The transverse colon may be felt across the umbilical region and the sigmoid colon is felt in the left iliac fossa. The caecum is often palpable in the right iliac fossa. The ascending and descending colons pass through the right and left lumbar regions respectively. Other normal organs which may be palpable are the aorta in the umbilical region, and a full urinary bladder or pregnant uterus rising out of the pelvis into the suprapubic region. Palpation of the umbilicus with the tip of the finger may reveal a circular defect in the linear alba. This is usually insignificant, but larger defects may transmit viscera producing an umbilical hernia with a cough impulse.

The lower pole of a normal right kidney may be palpated and this is felt by backward pressure of the flat of the right hand in the right lumbar region, combined with forward pressure from the left hand placed behind the abdomen, opposite the right hand. The kidney descends on inspiration and can be felt between the two hands in this bimanual palpation. For bimanual examination of the left lumbar region, the right hand is applied across the anterior abdomen in the usual fashion, and the left hand is either crossed behind the back of the subject with the examiner kneeling or placed behind the left lumbar region with the examiner leaning over the subject.

Percussion is used to define the lower borders of the liver and spleen, being undertaken along the defined lines of their enlarge-ment. The enlarged urinary bladder and uterus are dull to percus-sion as are abdominal masses and fluid within the peritoneal cavity. The latter is known as ascites and produces dullness in the flanks in the supine position. If the subject then rolls onto one side, the upper dull area will become resonant due to shifting of the fluid by gravity, a feature known as shifting dullness.

Bowel sounds can be heard with a stethoscope over all the abdomen. After a meal they are loudest and most frequent, but at other times it may be necessary to wait for a minute to hear them. Turbulence in the abdominal aorta or iliac vessels may produce sounds detectable with a stethoscope.

INGUINAL REGION, PERINEUM, SCROTUM AND PENIS

The aponeurotic lower border of the external oblique muscle (Fig. 5.2, p. 42) between the anterior superior iliac spine and the pubic tubercle is rolled back on itself to form a firm edge, the inguinal ligament. Just above and medial to the pubic tubercle there is an oval defect in the aponeurosis of the external oblique known as the superficial inguinal ring. In the male it forms the external opening of the canal in the abdominal wall through which the testis passes en route to the scrotum. The ring admits the tip of a little finger; it may be difficult to palpate in an obese subject and, alternatively, the tip of the finger can invaginate the skin of the scrotum upwards, behind the subcutaneous fat into the ring. The inguinal canal starts at a round opening in the transversalis fascia, the deep inguinal ring. This is not palpable but is situated about 1 cm above the middle of the inguinal ligament.

The femoral artery is found deep to the ligament at the mid-inguinal point (midway between the anterior superior iliac spine and the symphysis pubis). The inferior epigastric artery ascends medially from this point, medial to the deep ring. The femoral vein lies medial to the artery, within a common sheath. An areo-lar channel medial to the vein, allowing its expansion, forms the medial compartment of the sheath and contains fat, a few deep inguinal lymph nodes and the ascending lymphatic channels; it is termed the femoral canal (Fig. 8.7, p. 98). The sheath merges with the adventitia of the vessels at the level of the saphenous

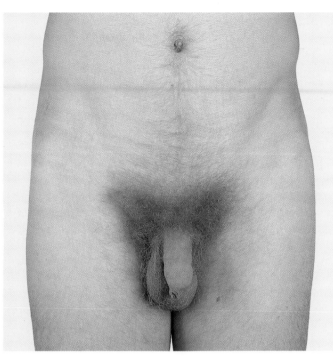

5.13
Inguinal region

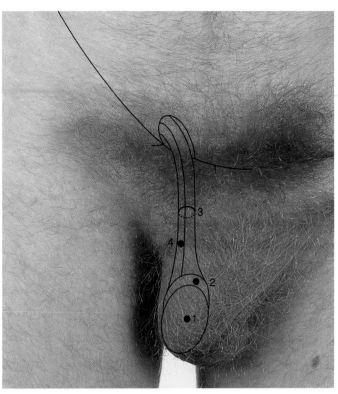

5.15
Testis and spermatic cord

1 Testis	3 Spermatic cord
2 Superior pole of epididymis	4 Vas deferens

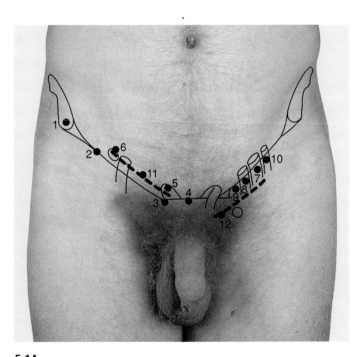

5.14
Inguinal region: bones and soft tissues

1 Anterior superior iliac spine	7 Femoral artery
2 Inguinal ligament	8 Femoral vein
3 Pubic tubercle	9 Femoral canal
4 Symphysis pubis	10 Femoral nerve
5 Superficial inguinal ring	11 Inguinal hernia incision
6 Deep inguinal ring	12 Femoral hernia incision

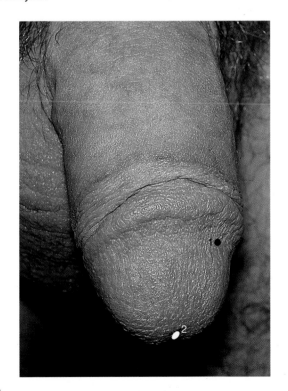

5.16
Penis
Compare this circumcised penis with that of Fig. 5.13, where the foreskin is intact

1 Glans penis	2 Urethral opening

opening, where the saphenous vein pierces the deep fascia to drain into the femoral vein.

Testicular descent draws a sac of peritoneum with the testicular vessels into the scrotum and the lower end of this sac surrounds the organ.

The communication with the peritoneal cavity usually closes off, but if it remains patent, peritoneal contents may pass into the sac along the length of the inguinal canal and into the scrotum; this condition is known as an indirect inguinal hernia. Gut may also bulge through a weak posterior wall of the inguinal canal medial to the inferior epigastric artery and protrude through the superficial inguinal ring; this is termed a direct inguinal hernia. A large inguinal hernia can be easily felt, particularly if the subject stands up and coughs. For small hernias, the tip of the little finger is introduced into the superficial inguinal ring as described above and will detect a cough impulse. Although the inguinal canal is rudimentary in the female, both forms of inguinal hernia may occur. Occasionally a peritoneal sac can be protruded into the femoral canal and emerge through the saphenous opening. This is known as a femoral hernia. The incisions shown in Figure 5.14 are used to approach inguinal and femoral hernias, removing the abnormal peritoneal sac and repairing the defect in the abdominal wall.

Scrotum and penis

The normal testis can be gently palpated through the walls of the scrotum, together with the upper and lower poles of the epididymis (Fig. 5.15). The vas (ductus) deferens ascends from the lower pole, posterior to the testis and can be palpated up to the superficial inguinal ring, rolling the cord-like structure between finger and thumb. The lower end of the peritoneal sac, drawn into the scrotum during testicular descent and surrounding the testis, normally contains a film of lubricant fluid within it.

If excessive fluid is produced, which may be related to a disease process, the condition is known as a hydrocele. The body of the penis ends in the expanded glans penis containing the external opening of the urethra. The skin over the glans, the prepuce (foreskin), is the tissue removed in circumcision. It is usually retractable after the age of 3 or 4 but may contract circumferentially over the end of the glans or, if then retracted, forms a constriction proximal to the glans; this condition is known as a paraphimosis. Examination of the scrotum, its contents and the penis should be a routine part of every full examination of a male patient, confirming a normal testis, epididymis and vas deferens bilaterally, and a normal penis.

5 FEMALE PERINEUM

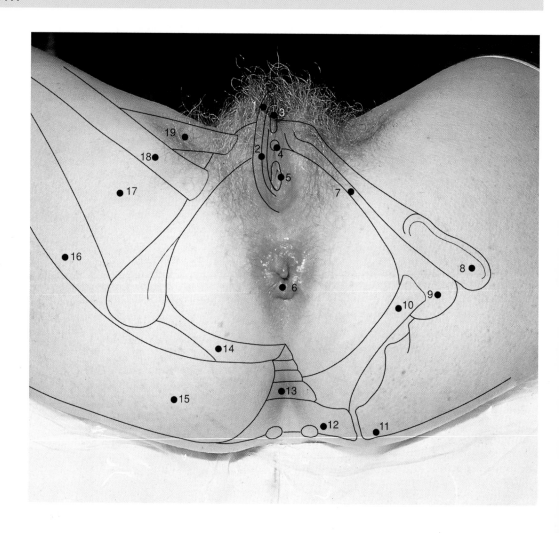

5.17
Female perineum
1 Labium majora
2 Labium minora
3 Clitoris
4 Urethral opening
5 Vaginal opening
6 Anus
7 Inferior pubic ramus
8 Acetabulum
9 Ischial tuberosity
10 Sacrotuberous ligament
11 Posterior inferior iliac spine
12 Sacrum
13 Coccyx
14 Sacrospinous ligament
15 Gluteus maximus
16 Hamstring muscles
17 Adductor magnus
18 Gracilis
19 Adductor longus

The opening of the vagina (the introitus) is surrounded by two labial (majora and minora) folds on each side. The labia majora unite anterosuperiorly around the clitoris, the embryological equivalent of the penis. The urethra opens between the clitoris and the vagina. The anus is situated in the midline, anterior to the coccyx and in line with the ischial tuberosities. The pelvic contents can be palpated with a gloved finger passed per rectum or vaginam (PR or PV). In digital examination of the rectum, the patient is usually lying on her left side on the edge of a couch, the examiner standing behind her back. On insertion of the right index finger, the examiner assesses the tone of the anal sphincter. Posteriorly is found the curve of the sacrum. The coccyx can be felt between the inserted finger and the thumb resting superficially, and laterally the ischial spines and tuberosities. In the male, the posterior aspect of the prostate gland can be palpated anteriorly and at a higher level, through the anterior rectal wall, the contents of the rectovesical pouch. The contents usually are loops of sigmoid colon and small gut, and sometimes the tip of the appendix.

Vaginal examination allows palpation of the cervix and, by pressing the left hand over the suprapubic region, bimanual examination usually enables the size and position of the uterus to be assessed. Ovaries lying on the broad ligament may also be palpable and the contents of the recto-uterine pouch (of Douglas) may be noted. Although such examinations are not necessarily very acceptable to clinician or patient, they can elicit important information about pelvic viscera. A PR is an essential part of every full clinical examination and a PV when obstetric or gynaecological conditions are being considered.

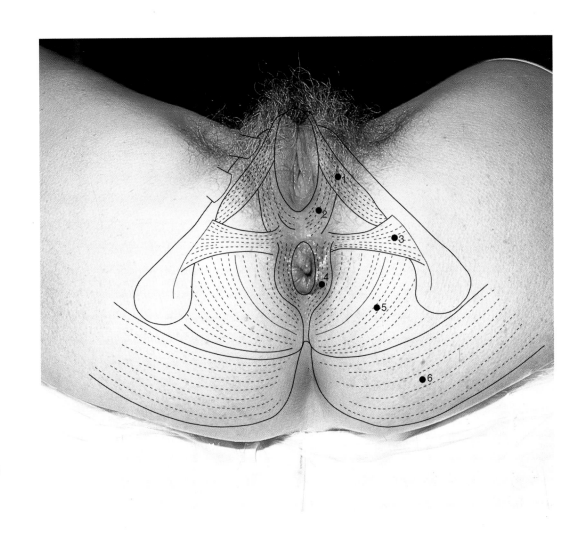

5.18
Muscles of female perineum
1 Ischiocavernosus
2 Bulbospongiosus
3 Transversus perinei superficialis
4 Sphincter ani externus
5 Levator ani
6 Gluteus maximus

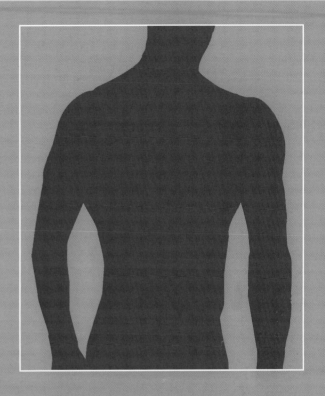

6

The *axial skeleton* is made up of the *skull* (pp. 10 and 12), the *spine* and the *rib cage* (p. 32). The spine (vertebral column) is an osseocartilaginous structure lying posteriorly in the midline. It articulates with the skull superiorly and extends through the neck and trunk to the tip of the coccyx. It articulates with the rib cage, forms part of the pelvis and gives attachment to the muscles of the shoulder girdle. The column thus provides a rigid, yet flexible, axis for the head to pivot; the upper limbs to be suspended and carry loads; the thoracic cage to be attached and function as an expansile respiratory unit; and the transfer of the body weight to the legs, when standing and in locomotion, and to the ischeal tuberosities when seated. The column also provides a protective covering for the spinal cord.

The vertebral column is made up of 33 vertebrae – seven cervical, 12 thoracic, five lumbar, five sacral and four coccygeal. Of these, 24 are mobile: the sacral vertebrae are fused and the coccygeal vestigial. The mobile vertebrae are united by fibrocartilaginous intervertebral discs, each comprising an outer firm ring, the annulus fibrosus, and a central gelatinous nucleus pulposus. The discs make up a quarter of the height of the column.

The embryonic and early fetal vertebral column is curved, concave ventrally (flexed) throughout its length – the primary curvature. Two secondary curvatures, concave dorsally, develop in the cervical and lumbar regions. The cervical curve starts as early as the 10th week 'in utero'. After birth, further extension in the cervical region is produced by the muscles raising the head, and extension in the lumbar region accompanies the adoption of the erect posture. The thoracic and sacral regions retain the primary curvature (Figs 6.1 and 6.2).

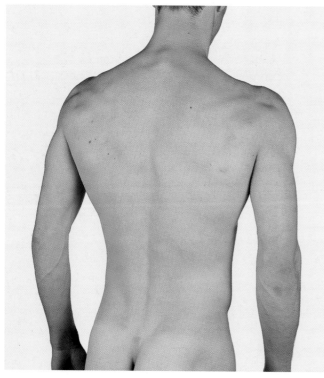

6.1
Spinal curvatures

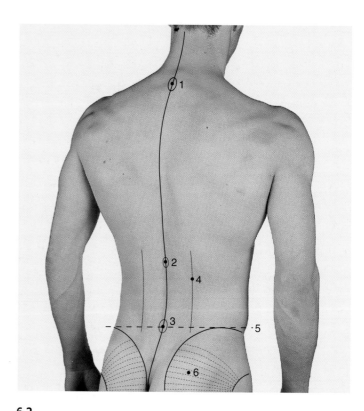

6.2
Spinal curvatures

1 Spine of first thoracic vertebra
2 Spine of twelfth thoracic vertebra
3 Spine of fourth lumbar vertebra
4 Lateral margin of erector spinae muscles
5 Intertubercular plane
6 Gluteus maximus

POSTERIOR ASPECT OF THE NECK

The posterior aspect of the neck is bounded superiorly by the superior nuchal line of the occipital bone extending medially to the external occipital protuberance and laterally to the mastoid process (Figs 6.3–6.5).

The structures in the lower part of the neck are less easily discernible posteriorly as they are covered by the trapezius, splenius and powerful erector spinae muscles. The ligamentum nuchae lies in the midline between the muscles of the two sides, and is attached to the occipital bone and the cervical spines. The spines of the lower two or three cervical, and all the thoracic, vertebrae are palpable. The upper cervical spines are impalpable and overlain by a median furrow. The non-bifed lowest (seventh) cervical vertebral spine and the first thoracic are the most obvious, the former being termed the vertebra prominens.

The trapezius muscle has a wide attachment (Figs 6.6 and 6.7, see also p. 68). It lies superficially and is attached superiorly to

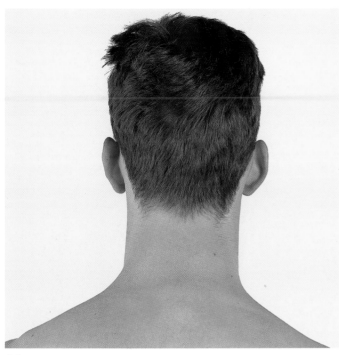

6.3
Posterior aspect of the neck

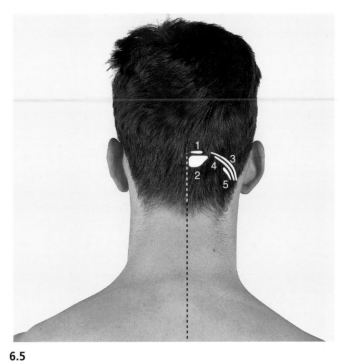

6.5
Posterior aspect of the neck: muscle attachments
1 Trapezius
2 Semispinalis capitis
3 Sternocleidomastoid
4 Splenius capitis
5 Superior oblique

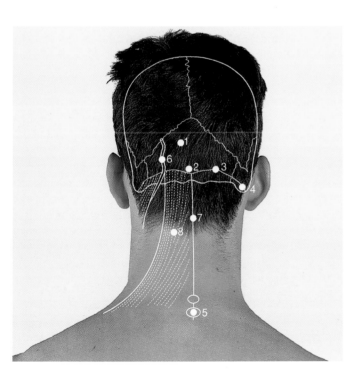

6.4
Posterior aspect of the neck: bones and soft tissues
1 Occipital bone
2 External occipital protuberance (inion)
3 Superior nuchal line
4 Mastoid process
5 Spine of first thoracic vertebra
6 Occipital artery
7 Ligamentum nuchae
8 Trapezius muscle

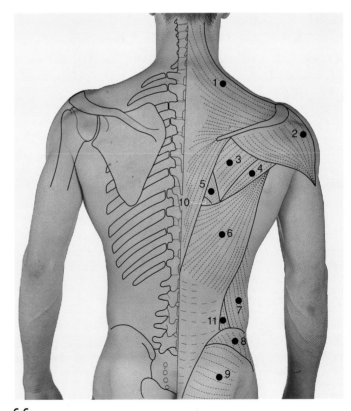

6.6
Posterior trunk: bones and superficial muscles
1 Trapezius
2 Deltoid
3 Infraspinatus
4 Teres major
5 Rhomboideus major
6 Latissimus dorsi
7 External oblique
8 Gluteus medius
9 Gluteus maximus
10 Auscultatory triangle
11 Lumbar triangle

the medial third of the superior nuchal line, to the ligament nuchae and the spines and interspinous ligaments of the cervical and thoracic vertebrae. Laterally, it is attached to the acromion and spine of the scapula, both of which are palpable from the tip of the shoulder to the medial angle of the bone. The sternocleidomastoid muscle is attached to the lateral third of the superior nuchal line and to the mastoid process. The occipital artery emerges medial to the muscle to pass over the skull; it is palpable at this site.

The superior nuchal line overlies the transverse venous sinus. The hindbrain lies below this level within the posterior fossa. The attachments of the trapezius, erector spinae and short occipital muscles have to be scraped off the surface of the occipital bone to allow surgical access to the posterior fossa. The vertebral artery lies deep to these muscles, crossing the suboccipital triangle.

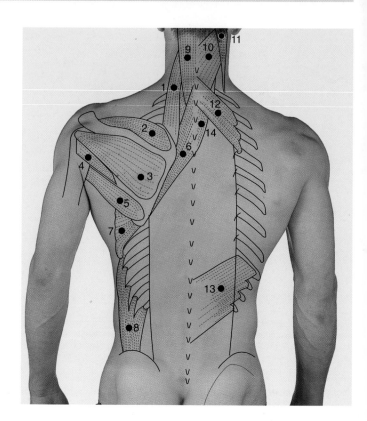

6.7
Posterior trunk: deep muscles of shoulder girdle

1 Levator scapulae	8 External oblique
2 Supraspinatus	9 and 14 Semispinalis capitis
3 Infraspinatus	
4 Teres minor	10 Splenius capitis
5 Teres major	11 Sternocleidomastoid
6 Rhomboid muscles	12 Serratus posterior superior
7 Serratus anterior	13 Serratus posterior inferior

POSTERIOR ASPECT OF THE TRUNK

The thoracic vertebrae give attachment to the 12 pairs of ribs making up the rib cage (p. 32), and the muscles of the shoulder girdle (p. 68). The free ends of the floating ribs and the costal margins are palpable, but most of the ribs cannot be felt through the muscle mass or the scapula that overlies the second to seventh ribs; these levels equate, respectively, to the body of the fourth (spine of the third) and ninth (spine of the eighth) thoracic vertebrae. The downward projecting thoracic spines are all palpable; counting is facilitated by asking the subject to bend forwards, when they jut out slightly. The lowest thoracic and all of the lumbar spines are horizontal and easily palpable. A precise landmark at this level is the spine of L4, which is in the inter-cristal plane, i.e. the line through the crests of the iliac bones (Fig. 6.2).

The spines of the sacrum, sacral hiatus and coccyx are usually palpable, curving anteriorly, and their anterior surface can be felt on rectal examination. The sacrum forms part of the pelvis, uniting with the ilium of each side through the sacroiliac joints which, although synovial, are immobile and often fused. The crest of the ilium is palpable from the anterior superior iliac spine throughout its length to the posterior superior iliac spine, which is overlain by a skin dimple. The posterior inferior iliac spine and the sacroiliac joints may also be palpable and, through the gluteus maximus, the posterior aspect of the acetabulum. Interiorly, the ischial tuberosities take the weight of the body when seated.

The female pelvis is relatively wider, has greater capacity, and its bones are thinner, smoother and lighter than those of the male. Other comparative features are a shallower acetabulum, a more vertical ilium, and a triangular rather than an oval-shaped obturator foramen; in addition, the width of the acetabulum is less than the distance from its anterior rim to the symphysis pubis, this distance being greater in the male. The inferior pubic angle is wider in the female.

STRUCTURE AND MOVEMENT OF THE VERTEBRAL COLUMN

The stability of the vertebral column is provided by the shape of the bones, including the curvatures, their intervertebral joints, strong ligaments and powerful muscles. The intervertebral discs act as shock absorbers between the short cylindrical vertebral bodies, conveying a certain resilience to the column.

Typical vertebrae have a body and a posterior bony arch; the body lies anteriorly, with a short stout pedicle on each side, completed posteriorly by the lamina, with a posterior projecting midline spine. The facets for the intervertebral synovial joints are sited at the junction of each pedicle and the lamina. The facets vary in shape in different regions, and this determines the type and amount of movement. Although the movement between adjacent vertebrae is small, a considerable range of movement is present in the vertebral column as a whole (Fig. 6.8). Flexion is

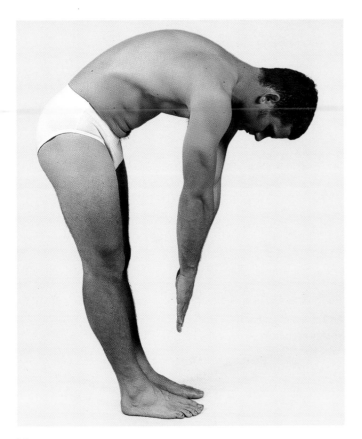

6.8
Spinal flexion

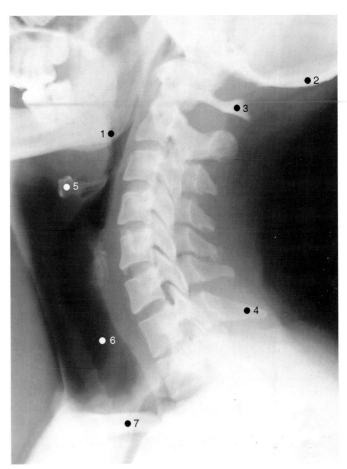

6.10
Cervical spine: lateral view
1 Angle of mandible
2 Occipital bone
3 Posterior arch of atlas
4 Spine of seventh
  cervical vertebra
5 Hyoid bone
6 Tracheal gas shadow
7 Clavicle

6

most marked in the cervical region, rotation in the thoracic region, and extension and lateral flexion in the lumbar region.

The first (atlas) and the second (axis) cervical vertebrae are atypical. The axis is an oval ring of bone articulating with the condyles of the occipital bone superiorly (facilitating head flexion and extension) and the horizontal flat atlantoaxial facets inferiorly, allowing rotation of the head on the neck. The body of the atlas has become fused with the axis to produce a process (the dens) separate from its origin and acting as a pivot around which the atlas rotates (Figs 6.9 and 6.10). The movement between the remaining cervical vertebrae is predominantly flexion and extension. Some lateral flexion is present and accompanied by slight

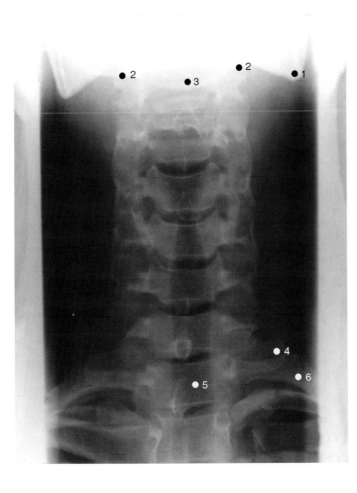

6.9
Cervical spine: anterior view
1 Mastoid process
2 Base of skull
3 Posterior arch of atlas
4 Transverse process of
  first thoracic vertebra
5 Body of first thoracic
  vertebra
6 First rib

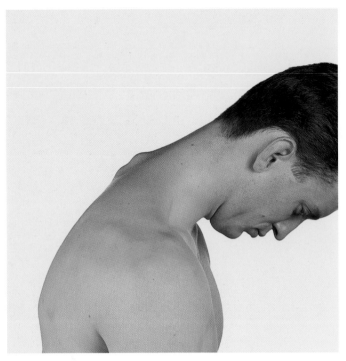

6.11
Neck flexion

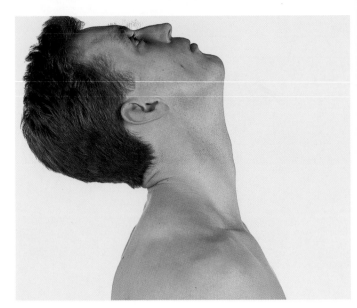

6.13
Neck extension

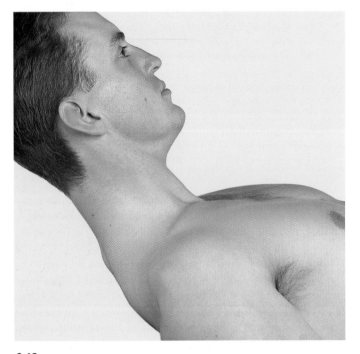

6.12
Raising the head from the horizontal

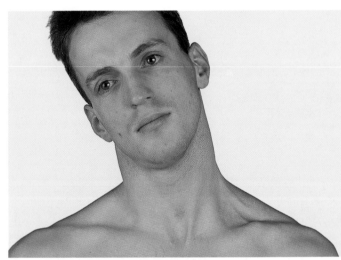

6.14
Lateral flexion of the neck

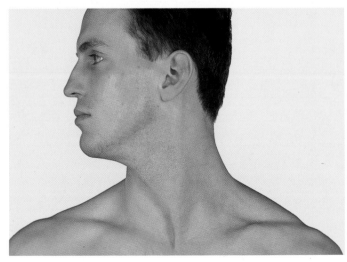

6.15
Lateral rotation of the neck

rotation. Head and neck movements are demonstrated in Figures 6.11–6.16.

Movement of the thoracic spine is limited by the rib cage and by the need for uninhibited respiratory movements. Some rotation is present, particularly between the lower thoracic vertebrae (Fig. 6.17). Movement of the lumbar spine is restricted to flexion and extension (Figs 6.18 and 6.19). This can be demonstrated by marking the lumbar spines and seeing their longitudinal

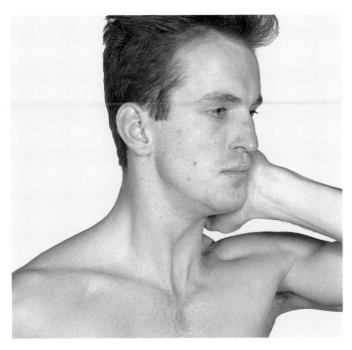

6.16
Resisted lateral rotation of the neck
Rotation is brought about by contraction of the right sternocleidomastoid muscle

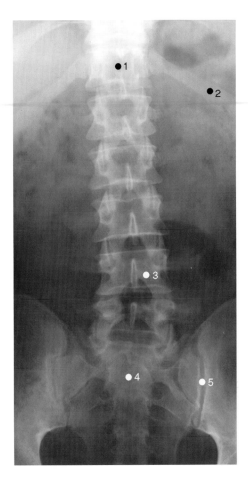

6.18
Lumbar spine: anterior view
1 Body of twelfth thoracic vertebra
2 Twelfth rib
3 Body of fourth lumbar vertebra
4 Sacrum
5 Sacroiliac joint

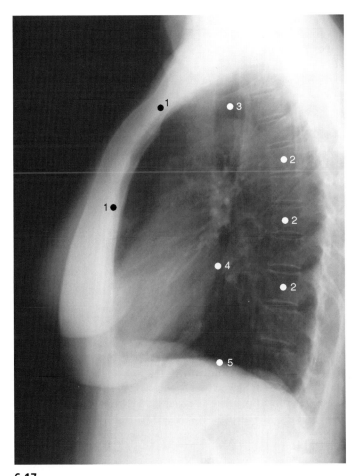

6.17
Thoracic spine: lateral view
1 Sternum
2 Bodies of thoracic vertebrae
3 Tracheal gas shadow
4 Posterior border of heart
5 Dome of diaphragm

separation when the subject is asked to touch his or her toes (Figs 6.20 and 6.21).

In the trunk, flexion is brought about by the rectus abdominis, aided by the prevertebral muscles. Lateral flexion is by the oblique abdominal wall muscles and quadratus lumborum, and rotation by the internal and external oblique abdominal muscles. The body's centre of gravity lies anterior to the second piece of the sacrum. Movement of the body frequently carries the centre of gravity much further forward and a large powerful posterior muscle mass is required both to balance the effects of gravity and to restore the upright position. This is primarily by the erector spinae muscles.

The erector spinae (sacrospinalis) is a large muscle mass on each side of the vertebral column, extending from the sacrum to the skull. It is a collective term for many small muscle groups passing between adjacent vertebrae or across a number of vertebrae. It varies in bulk at different levels. In the sacral region it is relatively narrow, predominantly tendinous and of great strength. The most prominent part is in the lumbar region, and its cylindrical form is visible and palpable. In the thoracic region the mass flattens out, extending laterally the angle of the ribs, to

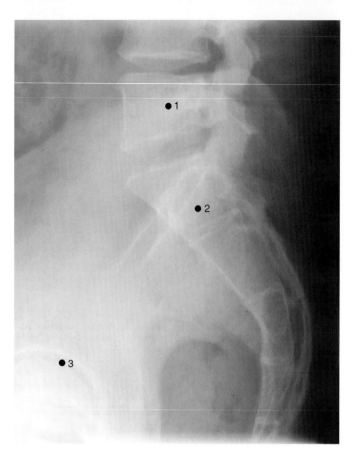

6.19
Lumbar spine: lateral view

1 Body of fifth lumbar vertebra	2 Sacrum
	3 Hip joint

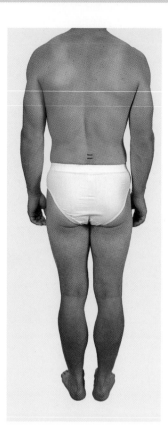

6.20
Posterior aspect of the lower trunk: at rest
The two skin marks are over the space between L3 and L4

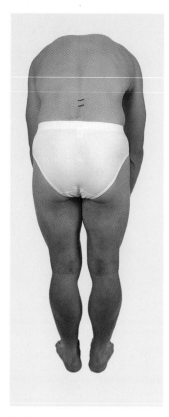

6.21
Lumbar flexion
The skin marks between L3 and L4 are stretched in relation to Fig. 6.20, but the palpable relation to the underlying spines has remained the same, demonstrating the contribution of the lumbar spine to trunk flexion

which it is also attached; it is covered by the scapula and muscles of the shoulder girdle. In the cervical region the cylindrical masses are covered by the trapezius and splenius muscles. Although three parallel columns can be identified in each erector spinae muscle, it is best considered as a powerful extensor unit acting on the vertebral column and the skull (Figs 6.22 and 6.23).

The lower lumbar vertebrae and discs, particularly the lumbosacral disc, are subject to the greatest load, stresses and strains. Musculoskeletal injuries are common in this region, resulting in low back pain. Degenerative changes in the annulus fibrosus allow protrusion of the nuclear content of a disc, with resultant pressure on adjacent tissues, such as the spinal cord or spinal nerves – the so-called 'prolapsed' (slipped) disc. Neurological signs may be present, together with spasm of the erector spinae muscles. Other clinical features are reduced spinal movement and loss of the normal lumbar lordosis.

Unilateral spasm causes scoliosis (lateral curvature in the coronal plain). Acute scoliosis of this form is usually compensated for by a compensatory curve in the thoracic region, the head and shoulders being maintained in line with the pelvis. Scoliosis is best observed from behind; it is made more obvious when the subject leans forward. Abnormalities of the spine may also produce lordosis and kyphosis – a concavity anteriorly and posteriorly, respectively, in the sagittal plain. In view of the fixed nature of the thoracic cage, scoliosis is usually accompanied by some rotation, producing a kyphoscoliotic spine.

Pain can be referred to the back from adjacent viscera. For example, disease of the descending thoracic aorta, such as rupture or dissection of an aneurysm, produces severe pain between the scapulae; in disease of the abdominal aorta, pain is projected to the lumbar region. Pancreatic disease produces central upper lumbar pain and the gall bladder right-sided pain at a similar level. Renal pain is characteristically in the subcostal region posteriorly. Pelvic disease, such as gynaecological infection and lower rectal pathology, can present with low back pain.

The muscle mass protects the abdominal viscera and lungs from injury, but major trauma can fracture ribs (putting the lungs, spleen and liver at risk) and damage the kidneys lying on the posterior abdominal wall.

Collectively, the arches of the vertebrae, together with their ligaments, and the vertebral bodies anteriorly form a longitudinal cylindrical cavity – the vertebral canal – that houses and protects the spinal cord and its coverings. There are eight pairs of cervical spinal nerves; the number at other levels is the same as the number of vertebrae. The upper seven cervical nerves leave the vertebral canal through intervertebral foramina above the pedicles of the equivalent vertebrae. The eighth cervical nerve passes beneath the pedicle of the seventh cervical vertebra. The thoracic and lumbar spinal nerves pass beneath the pedicles of the equivalent vertebrae. The sacral nerves pass out through foramina in the fused bone, and the coccygeal nerves pass through the sacral hiatus to the perineum.

The spinal cord finishes at the level of the third lumbar vertebra at birth, and the first lumbar vertebra in the adult. The disparity of length of the spinal cord and the vertebral canal means that caudal nerves descend an increasing distance within the meningeal coverings. The dural sac extends to the second sacral

vertebra. The collection of nerves below the spinal cord is known as the cauda equina. This anatomical arrangement has important clinical significance, since a needle can be introduced into the dural sac below the level of L3 in a baby and L1 in an adult without risk of damaging the spinal cord (Fig. 6.23). As noted, the fourth lumbar spine is in the intercristal plane – a needle is inserted above or below this spine in the procedure known as a lumbar puncture. It can be used to remove samples of cerebrospinal fluid, or introduce local anaesthetic into the extradural space, or dural sac, known, respectively, as epidural and spinal anaesthesia.

Injection of local anaesthetic into the sacral hiatus anaesthetises the lower spinal nerves, especially those supplying the perineal region. This is termed caudal anaesthesia and can be used to reduce the pain of childbirth. The lumbar spine and spinal cord are approached surgically through a posterior midline incision centred over the appropriate vertebra. One or more spines and laminae are removed to facilitate access (laminectomy).

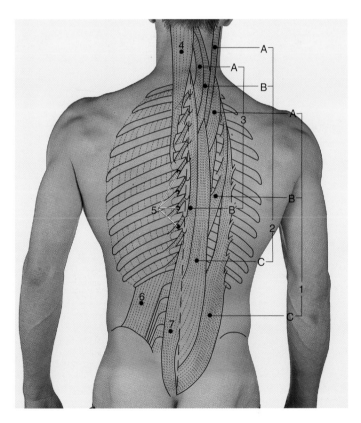

6.22
Posterior trunk: sacrospinalis
1 Iliocostalis
  A Cervicis
  B Thoracis
  C Lumborum
2 Longissimus
  A Capitis
  B Cervicis
  C Thoracis
3 Spinalis
  A Cervicis
  B Thoracis
4 Semispinalis capitis
5 Rotatores and levator costae
6 Quadratus lumborum
7 Multifidus

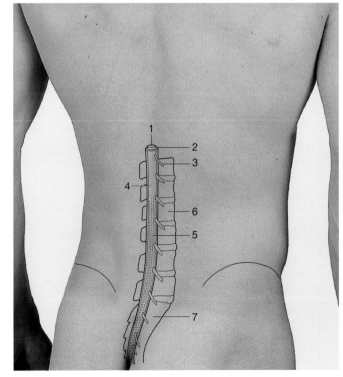

6.23
Spinal canal
1 Spinal cord
2 Dural sac
3 Spinal nerve
4 Conus medullaris
5 Cauda equina
6 Body of second lumbar vertebra
7 Sacrum

7 UPPER LIMB

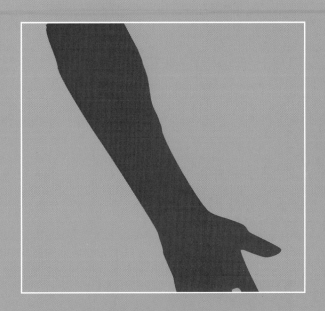

ANTERIOR ASPECT OF THE SHOULDER AND UPPER ARM

The shoulder girdle is the means by which the humerus of the upper limb is attached to the axial skeleton. It consists of the scapula and the clavicle (Fig. 7.2) and is supported by powerful proximal muscles.

Compression forces from the limb are transmitted through the humerus, scapula and clavicle to the axial skeleton. The clavicle articulates medially with the sternum and first rib at the sternoclavicular joint; the costoclavicular ligament is a powerful shock absorber. The clavicle articulates laterally with the scapula at the acromioclavicular joint and through strong coracoclavicular ligaments. The anterior surface of the clavicle, the acromion and the spine of the scapula are subcutaneous and palpable.

The lateral third of the clavicle, the acromion and the spine give lateral attachment to the trapezius muscle (Fig. 7.13, p. 69), which raises, laterally rotates and draws the scapula medially. It is supplied by the accessory (11th cranial) nerve. The deltoid muscle takes its medial attachments from the lateral quarter of the clavicle, the acromion and the spine of the scapula, and forms the smooth contour of the shoulder. Laterally, it is attached to the deltoid tubercle on the lateral aspect of the humerus. It is the prime abductor of the arm, its anterior fibres contributing to flexion and the posterior fibres to extension of the limb; it is supplied by the axillary nerve. The upper end of the humerus can be palpated through the fibres of the relaxed deltoid.

The pectoralis major muscle has two medial heads (Fig. 7.5). The clavicular is attached to the medial two-thirds of the clavicle and the sternocostal to the anterior surface of the sternum, the upper five to seven costal cartilages and the upper part of the external oblique aponeurosis. Laterally, the two heads converge onto a narrow tendon which passes deep to the deltoid muscle to be attached to the lateral lip of the bicipital groove on the humerus. The superior head overlaps the inferior and together they form the bulk of the anterior axillary fold (Fig. 4.12, p. 38). The muscle as a whole is a powerful abductor and medial rotator of the arm; the clavicular head, with the anterior fibres of deltoid, flexes the arm. In contrast, the sternocostal head is a powerful

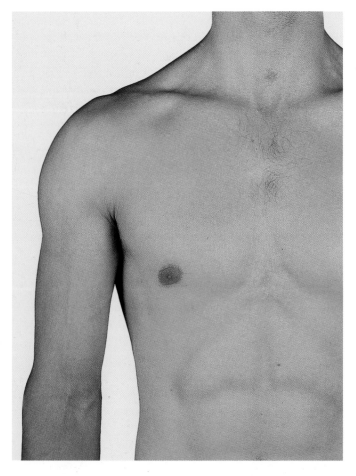

7.1
Anterior aspect of the shoulder and upper arm

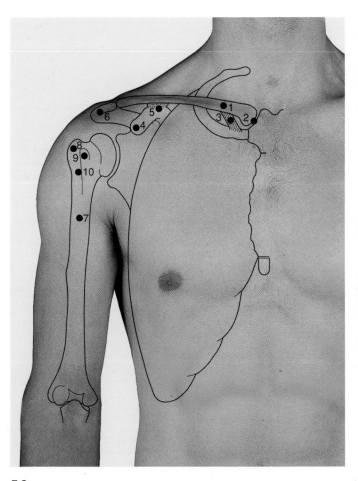

7.2
Anterior aspect of the shoulder and upper arm: bones

1 Clavicle	6 Acromion
2 Sternoclavicular joint	7 Humerus
3 Costoclavicular ligament	8 Greater tuberosity
4 Coracoid process	9 Lesser tuberosity
5 Coracoclavicular ligaments	10 Bicipital groove

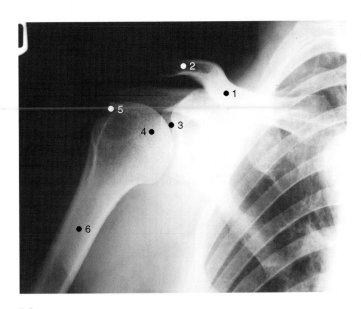

7.3

Anterior aspect of the shoulder

1 Clavicle
2 Acromion
3 Shoulder joint
4 Head of humerus
5 Greater tuberosity
6 Shaft of humerus

extensor from the flexed position, acting with latissimus dorsi (Fig. 7.13, p. 69), e.g. pulling the body up on an overhead bar and the follow-through of a tennis serve. It can be accentuated by pressing hands on hips (Fig. 7.6). The muscle is supplied by the medial and the lateral pectoral nerves from the brachial plexus.

The cephalic vein lies in the deltopectoral groove medial to the anterior fibres of the deltoid muscle. It passes deeply through the clavipectoral fascia (a layer between the pectoralis minor and the clavicle) to enter the axillary vein.

Falls onto the outstretched hand can result in fractures of the clavicle; this usually occurs at the junction of the middle and lateral thirds. Fractures of the humerus are usually by direct violence. At the upper end this is through the surgical neck; the axillary nerve is at risk as it lies adjacent to this site. Fractures of the humeral shaft are usually spiral, and the radial nerve, lying in its groove on the posterior aspect of the bone, is at risk; nerve injury produces wrist drop. The shoulder joint is least supported inferiorly, and dislocation is usually due to a blow to the upper lateral aspect of the abducted humerus. The axillary nerve is again at risk. Sensation should be assessed over the distal attachment of the deltoid, since this examination, of the upper lateral cutaneous branch of the axillary nerve, is less painful than testing the action of deltoid in the immediate post-traumatic period.

7.4

Anterior aspect of the shoulder and upper arm: muscle attachments

1 Pectoralis minor
2 and 11 Coracobrachialis
3 Short head of biceps
4 Long head of biceps
5 Long head of triceps
6 Supraspinatus
7 Subscapularis
8 Pectoralis major
9 Latissimus dorsi
10 Teres major
12 Deltoid
13 Brachialis

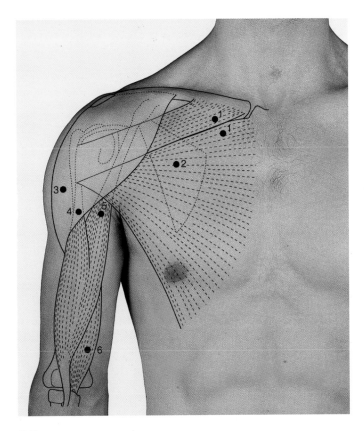

7.5

Anterior aspect of the shoulder and upper arm: muscles

1 Pectoralis major
2 Pectoralis minor
3 Deltoid
4 Long head of biceps
5 Short head of biceps
6 Brachialis

7

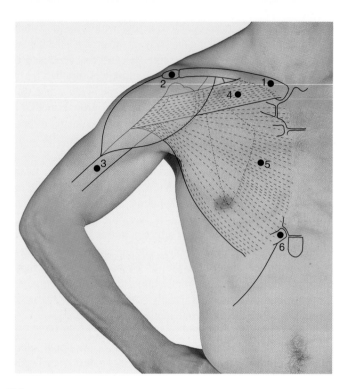

7.6
Action of the pectoralis major muscle

1 Clavicle
2 Acromion
3 Humerus
4 Pectoralis major clavicular head
5 Pectoralis major sternocostal head
6 Seventh costal cartilage

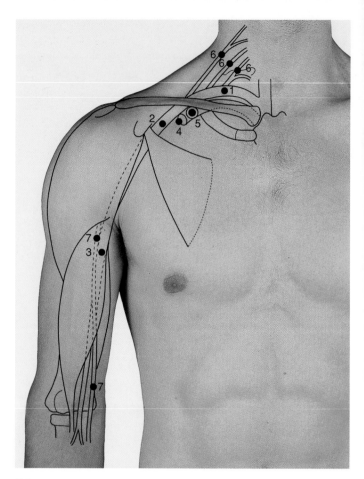

7.8
Anterior aspect of the shoulder and upper arm: vessels and nerves

1 Subclavian artery
2 Axillary artery
3 Brachial artery
4 Axillary vein
5 Site of access to subclavian vein
6 Brachial plexus: trunks separated for clarity
7 Median nerve

The axillary artery and vein can be exposed through an incision through skin and superficial fascia, separating the two heads of the pectoralis major muscle and dividing the clavipectoral fascia. The axillary vein becomes the subclavian vein at the outer border of the first rib behind the middle of the clavicle and is closely related to the posterior surface of this bone. A needle inserted below the clavicle and aimed superomedially adjacent to the posterior aspect of the bone will enter the vein; this provides an important point of access (Fig. 7.8).

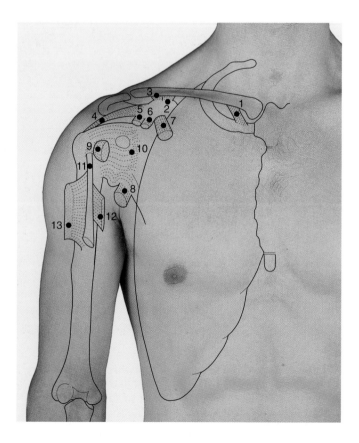

7.7
Shoulder joint: anterior aspect

1 Costoclavicular ligament
2 Conoid ligament
3 Trapezoid ligament
4 Coracohumeral ligament
5 Short head of biceps
6 Coracobrachialis
7 Pectoralis minor
8 Long head of triceps
9 Subscapularis
10 Anterior capsule of shoulder joint with opening of subscapular bursa
11 Long head of biceps
12 Latissimus dorsi
13 Pectoralis major

7

The brachial artery lies in the groove between the biceps and brachialis muscles along the length of the arm: it can be palpated by lateral pressure onto the humerus. The median nerve crosses anterior to the brachial artery in the mid-upper arm and comes to lie on its medial side in the cubital fossa. The shoulder joint may be approached through an anterior incision along the anterior border of the deltoid muscle, dividing its attachment to the clavicle and the tendon of the subscapularis muscle, to expose the capsule and anterior surface of the joint.

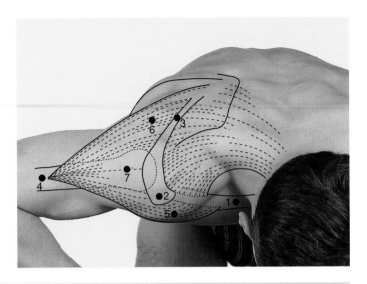

7.9
Attachments and action of the deltoid muscle

1 Clavicle	5 Anterior fibres
2 Acromion	6 Posterior fibres
3 Spine of the scapula	7 Lateral fibres
4 Humerus	

ACTIONS OF THE BICEPS MUSCLE

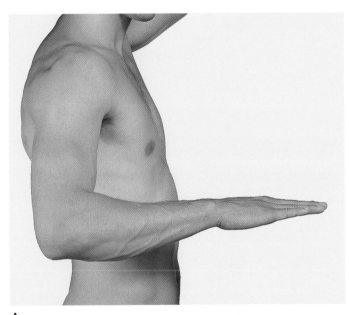

A

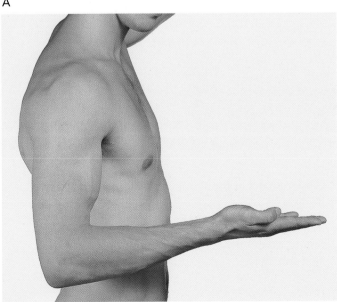

B

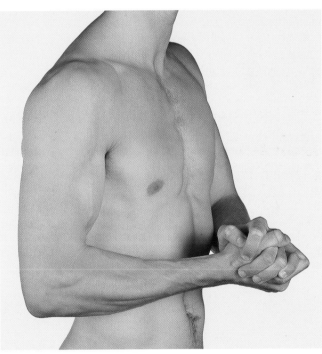

C

The tendon of the long head of the biceps muscle is palpable between the lesser and the greater tuberosities of the humerus. The coracoid process of the scapula gives attachment to the coracobrachialis, the short head of the biceps and the pectoralis minor muscles. It can be palpated deeply 1 cm below the clavicle under the medial fibres of the deltoid muscle.

The biceps muscle forms a prominence on the anterior aspect of the arm. Its short head is attached to the coracoid process and the long head passes between the greater and lesser humeral tuberosities, within the bicipital groove, and is attached to the superior

7.10
Actions of the biceps muscle
A, pronation; B, supination;
C, forced flexion and supination

7

aspect of the glenoid fossa on the scapula. Inferiorly the muscle is attached to the bicipital tuberosity on the radius; it has no attachments to the humerus. The muscle flexes the elbow and is a powerful supinator of the forearm: combining these actions produces the greatest prominence of the muscle belly (Fig. 7.10C). The muscle is supplied by the musculocutaneous nerve, which also supplies the coracobrachialis and brachialis muscles. The former muscle is not easily palpable in the lateral aspect of the axilla but the latter forms, with the biceps, the muscle bulk of the anterior aspect of the upper arm.

POSTERIOR ASPECT OF THE SHOULDER AND UPPER ARM

The acromion and spine of the scapula are subcutaneous. The deltoid muscle forms the smooth prominence of the shoulder overlapping the upper end of the humerus; its posterior fibres aid in extension of the shoulder (Fig. 7.13).

The trapezius forms a wide triangular muscle sheet with its base medially attached to the medial half of the superior nuchal line of the occipital bone, the ligamentum nuchae and the spines and interspinous ligaments of the lower cervical and all the thoracic vertebrae. Laterally the muscle is attached to the lateral third of the clavicle and to the length of the acromion and the spine of the scapula. The wide medial attachment of the muscle produces a wide range of scapular movements, raising, laterally rotating and drawing the bone medially (Figs 7.15–7.17). The muscle is supplied by the accessory (11th cranial) nerve.

The latissimus dorsi muscle also has a wide medial attachment, to the lumbar spines, lumbar fascia and posterior half of the iliac crest. Its fibres pass upwards and laterally to the floor of the bicipital groove on the humerus. The muscle is also attached to the inferior angle of the scapula, producing medial rotation, and helps to prevent this angle from jutting out from the chest wall during shoulder movements. The latissimus dorsi is a powerful adductor of the arm; its narrow tendon wraps around the teres major muscle in the posterior axillary wall. It is supplied by the thoracodorsal branch of the posterior cord of the brachial plexus, the nerve descending over the medial wall of the axilla to enter the muscle in the axilla.

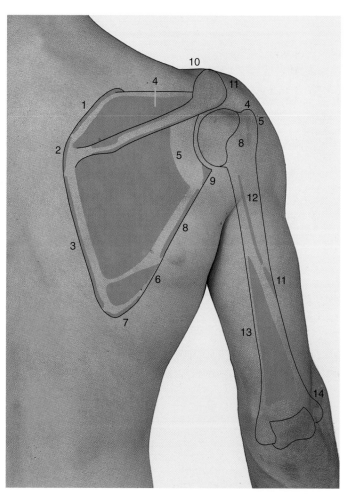

7.12
Posterior aspect of the shoulder and upper arm: muscle attachments

1 Levator scapulae	8 Teres minor
2 Rhomboideus minor	9 Long head of triceps
3 Rhomboideus major	10 Trapezius
4 Supraspinatus	11 Deltoid
5 Infraspinatus	12 Lateral head of triceps
6 Teres major	13 Medial head of triceps
7 Latissimus dorsi	14 Anconeus

7.11
Posterior aspect of the shoulder and upper arm

The lower part of the posterior axillary fold is formed mainly of the teres major muscle, passing from the dorsum of the inferior angle of the scapula to the medial lip of the bicipital groove on the humerus. The lateral border of the scapula can be felt through the bulk of the teres major muscle. The subscapularis muscle contributes to the posterior axillary wall superiorly. Together, the supraspinatus, infraspinatus, teres minor and subscapularis are termed the 'rotator cuff' muscles, being closely applied to the shoulder joint and maintaining its stability.

The teres major and the subscapularis muscles pass anterior to the joint, the latter to the lesser tuberosity, and are medial rotators of the shoulder joint. The infraspinatus and teres minor muscles pass posterior to the joint to the greater tuberosity and are lateral rotators. The former muscle is attached medially to the posterior aspect of the scapula below its spine and is palpable, the latter to its lateral border.

The supraspinatus muscle is attached to the posterior aspect of the scapula above the spine and is palpable deep to the trapezius. It passes laterally under the acromion to the greater tuberosity of the humerus. It also stabilises the shoulder joint and is important in initiating abduction, as the deltoid muscle has insufficient mechanical advantage to initiate this movement from the adducted position.

If the supraspinatus muscle is inactive the arm has to be swung or flicked by the hip laterally, away from the body, to enable the deltoid to take over abduction. While not primarily a rotator, supraspinatus does form one of the 'cuff' muscles.

The supraspinatus tendon is compressed between the greater tuberosity of the humerus and the acromion in mid-abduction; the arm has to be laterally rotated for full abduction to take place. This can be demonstrated by holding the medial and lateral epicondyles of the humerus through the full range of abduction. The supraspinatus and infraspinatus muscles are supplied by the suprascapular nerve from the upper trunk, and the teres major and suprascapularis muscles by the subscapular nerves from the posterior cord of the brachial plexus. All the intrinsic scapular muscles derive their nerve supply from the fifth and

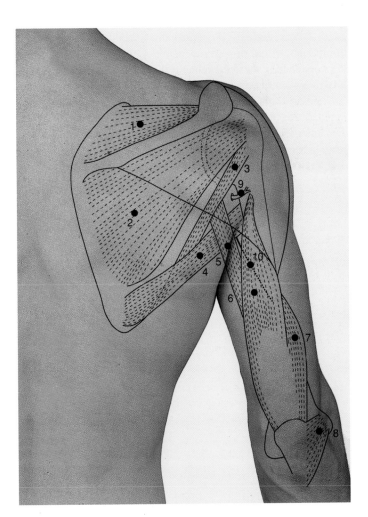

7.13
Posterior aspect of the shoulder and upper arm: bones and muscles of the shoulder girdle
Right, superficial muscles; left, deep muscles

1 Acromion	10 Deltoid
2 Spine of scapula	11 Latissimus dorsi
3 Medial border of scapula	12 Levator scapulae
4 Inferior angle of scapula	13 Rhomboideus minor
5 Medial angle of scapula	14 Rhomboideus major
6 Superior angle of scapula	15 Supraspinatus
7 Glenoid fossa	16 Infraspinatus
8 Humerus	17 Teres major
9 Trapezius	18 Teres minor

7.14
Posterior aspect of the shoulder and upper arm: structures deep to the deltoid muscle

1 Supraspinatus	6 Lateral head of triceps
2 Infraspinatus	7 Medial head of triceps
3 Teres minor	8 Anconeus
4 Teres major	9 Axillary nerve
5 Long head of triceps	10 Radial nerve

sixth cervical spinal nerve roots. The rotator muscles and supraspinatus stabilise the shoulder joint anteriorly, posteriorly and superiorly.

There is poor muscle support inferiorly and dislocation of the joint is usually in this direction. The axillary nerve supplies the deltoid muscle; it is closely applied to the neck of the humerus and may be damaged in this injury.

The muscle bulk of the posterior aspect of the upper arm is produced by the triceps muscle with a smaller contribution from the anconeus near the elbow (Fig. 7.14). The triceps is attached to the posterior shaft of the humerus above (lateral head) and below (medial head) the radial groove and, by its long head, below the glenoid fossa on the scapula. The muscle is attached distally to the palpable olecranon process of the ulna and is a powerful extensor of the elbow; it is supplied by the radial nerve.

This nerve runs obliquely, laterally across the humerus, close to the bone and may be injured in fractures of the humeral shaft with resultant paralysis of the extensor muscles of the forearm. The triceps is spared in this injury, as it is supplied from above this level.

MOVEMENTS OF THE SCAPULA AND SHOULDER JOINT

Movements of the upper limb away from the trunk involve movements both of the scapula and of the shoulder joint. This can be confirmed by watching a subject from behind and then trying to hold the scapula still during shoulder movements (Figs 7.15–7.17). Powerful muscles raise, lower, draw medially and laterally, and rotate the bone medially (medial movement of the inferior angle and downward facing of the glenoid fossa) and laterally. During these movements there is also some compensatory movement in the joints at either end of the clavicle.

The scapula is elevated, as in shrugging the shoulders, by the upper fibres of the trapezius and the levator scapulae muscles. The latter muscle lies deep to the trapezius and is attached to the medial border above the spine of the scapula and superiorly to the cervical transverse processes. It forms some of the muscle bulk of the posterolateral aspect of the neck. The scapula is depressed by the action of gravity and the serratus anterior and pectoralis minor muscles. The scapula is moved forwards on the chest wall, as in pushing and punching, by the serratus anterior and pectoralis minor muscles. The attachments of the latissimus dorsi to the inferior angle hold it onto the chest wall, but if the serratus anterior muscle is paralysed the inferior angle juts out during these movements, a condition known as winging of the scapula. Retraction of the scapula, as in bracing the shoulders, is by trapezius and, deep to this, the rhomboid muscles, passing between the medial aspect of the scapula and the thoracic spines. Lateral rotation of the scapula is produced by serratus anterior and trapezius, and medial rotation by levator scapulae, pectoralis minor and the rhomboid muscles.

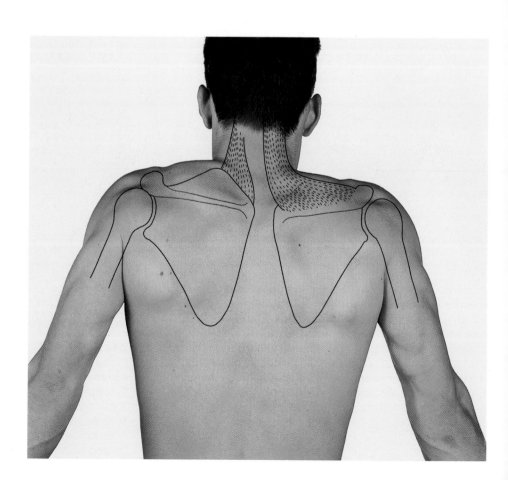

7.15
Scapula elevation

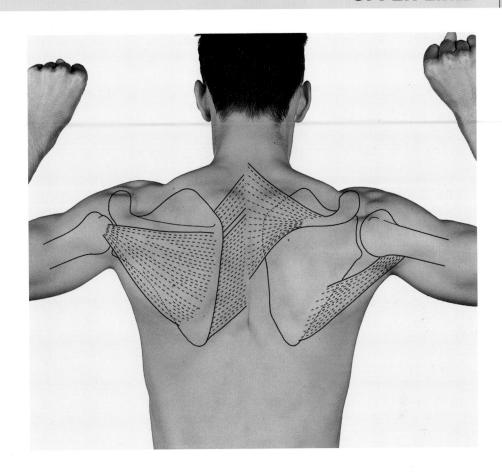

7.16
Scapula retraction

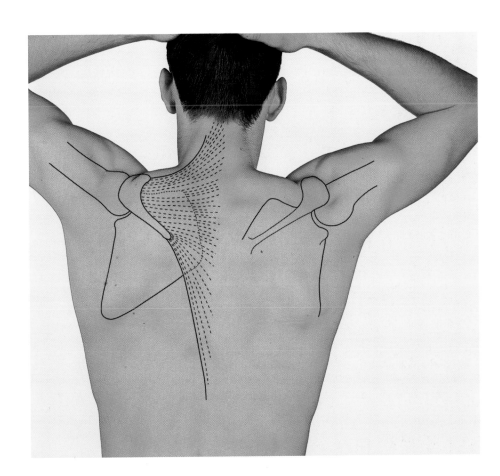

7

7.17
Lateral rotation of the
scapula

Flexion of the shoulder joint is by the clavicular head of the pectoralis major, the anterior fibres of the deltoid and coraco-brachialis muscles. Extension is by the posterior fibres of deltoid and, from the flexed position, by the sternocostal head of pectoralis major and latissimus dorsi muscles. Abduction is initiated by the supraspinatus and continued by the deltoid muscles. Medial rotation is by pectoralis major, the anterior fibres of deltoid and latissimus dorsi, teres major and subscapularis muscles. Lateral rotation is by the posterior fibres of deltoid, teres minor and the infraspinatus muscles.

CUBITAL FOSSA

The cubital fossa is bounded superiorly by a line through the palpable medial and lateral epicondyles of the humerus, laterally by the brachioradialis muscle and medially by the pronator teres muscle (Fig. 7.19). The brachialis muscle has a wide attachment to the anterior aspect of the humerus and its tendon passes to the coronoid process of the ulna in the floor of the cubital fossa, making it difficult to palpate the bones on the anterior aspect of the elbow joint. The prominent biceps tendon passes to the

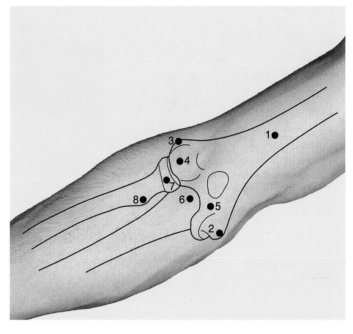

7.19
Cubital fossa: bones
1 Humerus
2 Medial epicondyle of humerus
3 Lateral epicondyle of humerus
4 Capitulum
5 Trochlea
6 Coronoid process of ulna
7 Head of radius
8 Bicipital tuberosity

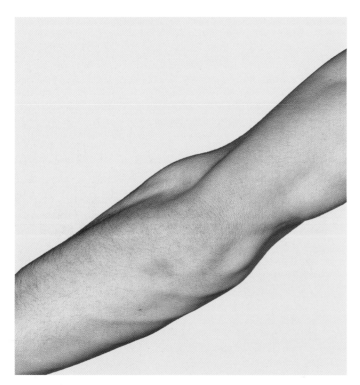

7.18
Cubital fossa and the anterior aspect of the forearm

7.20
Elbow joint

A, anterior
1 Shaft of humerus
2 Medial epicondyle
3 Trochlea, overlain by upper end of ulna
4 Capitulum
5 Head of radius
6 Shaft of radius
7 Shaft of ulna

B, lateral
1 Shaft of humerus
2 Head of radius
3 Coronoid process of ulna
4 Olecranon process of ulna

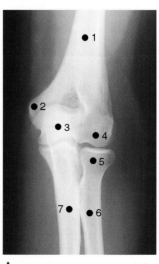

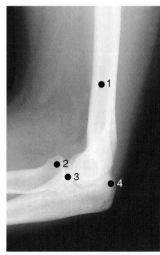

A

B

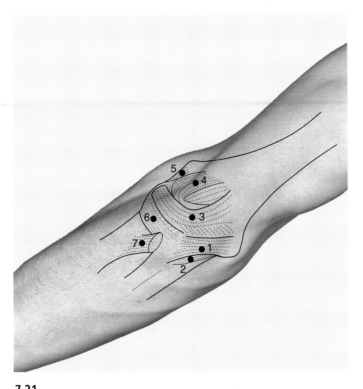

bicipital tuberosity, on the medial side of the upper end of the radius, through the middle of the fossa.

The firm thin bicipital aponeurosis passes from the medial side of the tendon in the roof of the fossa to the subcutaneous surface of the ulna (Fig. 7.22). The aponeurosis makes it more difficult to feel the brachial artery which has the median nerve lying on its medial side. To feel the artery, the elbow is fully extended and the vessel compressed back onto the joint; it passes deeply into the apex of the cubital fossa where it divides into the radial and ulnar arteries.

The brachial artery may be used to obtain an arterial blood sample or to insert catheters for cardiac and other arterial investigations. The median nerve leaves the fossa between the humeral and ulnar heads of pronator teres, and deep to the superficial muscles of the forearm. The cephalic, basilic and median cubital veins in the roof of the cubital fossa are commonly used for obtaining venous samples (Fig. 7.23).

7.21
Elbow joint: anterior aspect

1 Anterior band of medial ligament	3 and 4 Anterior capsule
2 Oblique band of medial ligament	5 Lateral ligament
	6 Annular ligament
	7 Tendon of biceps

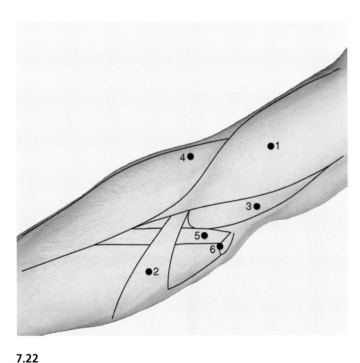

7.22
Cubital fossa: soft tissues

1 Biceps	4 Brachioradialis
2 Bicipital aponeurosis	5 Pronator teres
3 Brachialis	6 Common flexor origin

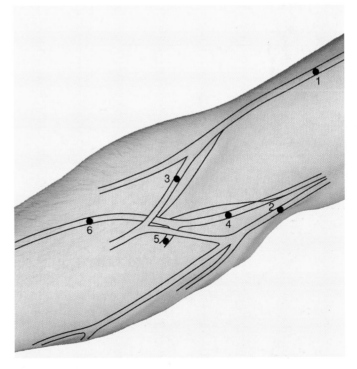

7.23
Cubital fossa: vessels

1 Cephalic vein	4 Brachial artery
2 Basilic vein	5 Ulnar artery
3 Median cubital vein	6 Radial artery

7

ANTERIOR ASPECT OF THE FOREARM

The pronator teres muscle is attached proximally just above the common flexor origin, on the anterior surface of the medial epicondyle. The common flexor origin gives attachment to the flexor carpi radialis, palmaris longus, flexor digitorum superficialis and flexor carpi ulnaris (Figs 7.26, 7.27 and 7.28). The pronator teres gains an additional head from the coronoid process of the ulna, and the flexor carpi ulnaris one from the posterior subcutaneous border of the bone; the former muscle is attached distally to the lateral aspect of the mid-shaft of the radius, and it pronates the forearm.

The tendons of the other common flexor origin muscles pass to the hand (Fig. 7.43, p. 81). These muscles are also weak flexors of the elbow: flexor carpi ulnaris is supplied by the ulnar nerve; the remainder by the median. The flexor pollicis longus, flexor digitorum profundus and, distally, the pronator quadratus muscles are deeply placed and impalpable in the forearm; all three are supplied by the anterior interosseus branch of the median nerve, the flexor digitorum profundus receiving an additional supply from the ulnar nerve (Fig. 7.28).

The brachoradialis muscle is attached proximally to the upper two-thirds of the lateral supracondylar ridge of the humerus and distally to the lateral aspect of the distal end of the radius; it pronates or supinates the forearm into the midprone position (flexion of the elbow joint is most powerful in this position). The muscle overlies the radial nerve and its posterior interosseous branch in the cubital fossa and is supplied by the former. The radial nerve also supplies the extensor carpi radialis longus muscle which is attached to the lower third of the lateral supracondylar ridge of the humerus; the muscle is deeply placed in the forearm but its tendon is palpable at the wrist (Fig. 7.51, p. 84).

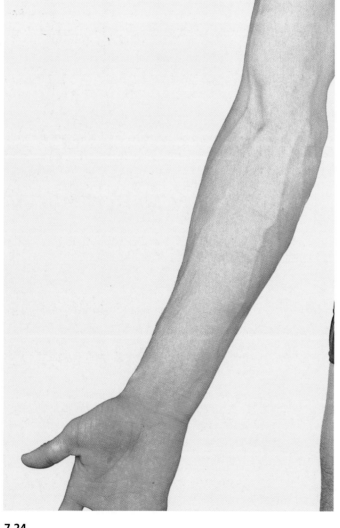

7.24
Anterior aspect of the forearm

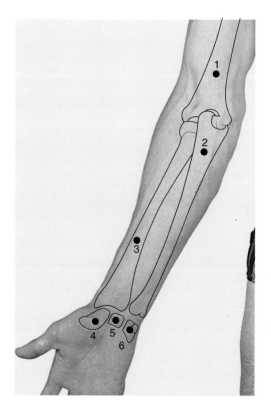

7.25
Anterior aspect of the forearm: bones

1 Humerus	4 Scaphoid
2 Ulna	5 Lunate
3 Radius	6 Triquetral

7.26
Anterior aspect of the forearm: muscle attachments
1 Brachioradialis
2 Extensor carpi radialis longus
3 Common extensor origin
4 and 13 Pronator teres
5 Common flexor origin
6 and 12 Flexor digitorum sublimus
7 Deep head of pronator teres
8 Brachialis
9 Flexor digitorum profundus
10 Biceps
11 Supinator
14 Flexor pollicis longus
15 Pronator quadratus

7.27
Anterior aspect of the forearm: superficial muscles
1 Pronator teres
2 Flexor carpi radialis
3 Palmaris longus
4 Flexor carpi ulnaris
5 Pisiform bone
6 Brachioradialis

7.28
Anterior aspect of the forearm: deep muscles
1 Tendon of biceps
2 Supinator
3 Flexor pollicis longus
4 Flexor digitorum profundus
5 Pronator quadratus

7.29
Flexor digitorum superficialis
1 Humero-ulnar head
2 Radial head
3 Tendons to middle and ring fingers lying anterior to those to the index and little fingers

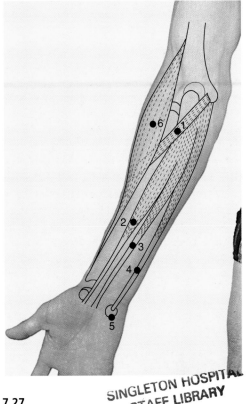

7.26

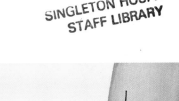
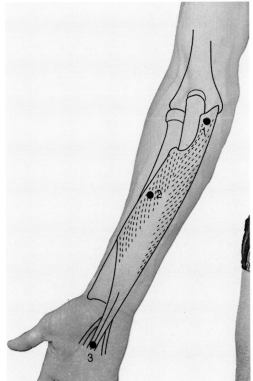

7.27

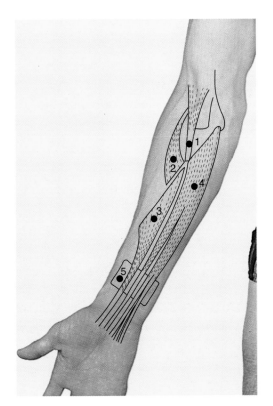

7.28

7.29

7

POSTERIOR ASPECT OF THE ELBOW AND FOREARM

The bones forming the elbow joint are more easily palpable posteriorly. The medial and lateral epicondyles can be grasped between finger and thumb and they are useful indicators of the position of the humerus in rotation of the shoulder joint (Fig. 7.31). The posterior border of the ulna is subcutaneous throughout its length. The triceps forms the main posterior muscle bulk of the upper arm and is attached to the palpable olecranon process. The head of the radius, ensheathed in the annular ligament, is palpable through the muscles attached to the common extensor origin on the posterior aspect of the lateral epicondyle. These muscles are the extensor carpi radialis brevis, extensor digitorum, extensor digiti minimi and extensor carpi ulnaris; they are weak extensors of the elbow joint and are supplied by the posterior interosseous nerve (Fig. 7.34).

The supinator is also attached to the common extensor origin at a deeper level and receives a head from the lateral aspect of the upper end of the ulna. The muscle wraps around the upper end of the radius to be attached to the anterior surface. It and the other deep impalpable muscles on the posterior aspect of the forearm are supplied by the posterior interosseous nerve; the tendons of these muscles are palpable at the wrist (Fig. 7.51, p. 84). The ulnar nerve lies posterior to the medial epicondyle and can be rolled over the bone at this point, before passing between the humeral and ulnar heads of the flexor carpi ulnaris. If knocked at this point it produces a pins and needles sensation in the forearm.

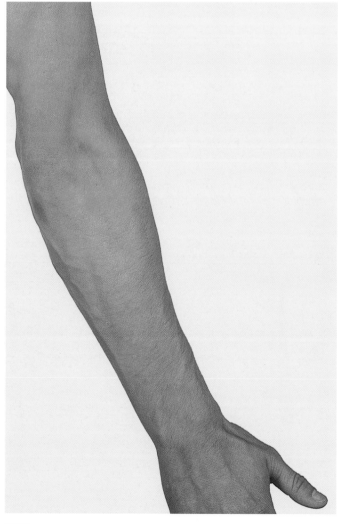

7.30
Posterior aspect of the elbow and forearm

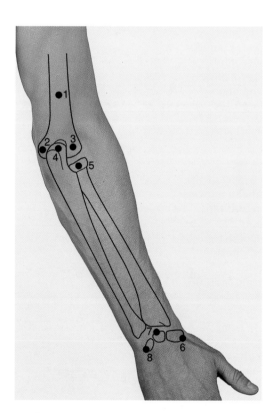

7.31
Posterior aspect of the elbow and forearm: bones

1 Humerus
2 Medial epicondyle of humerus
3 Lateral epicondyle of humerus
4 Olecranon process of ulna
5 Head of radius
6 Scaphoid
7 Lunate
8 Triquetral

7.32
Posterior aspect of the elbow and forearm: muscle attachments
1 Triceps
2 and 3 Anconeus
4 Posterior border of ulna giving attachment to extensor carpi ulnaris, flexor carpi ulnaris and flexor digitorum profundus
5 Biceps
6 Supinator
7 Abductor pollicis longus
8 Pronator teres
9 Extensor pollicis longus
10 Extensor pollicis brevis
11 Extensor indicis

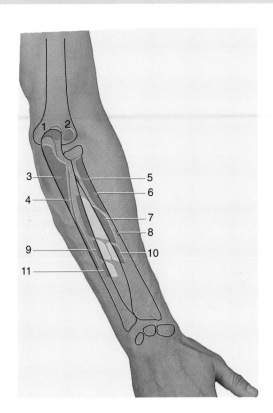

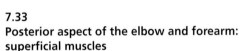

7.33
Posterior aspect of the elbow and forearm: superficial muscles
1 Brachioradialis
2 Extensor carpi radialis longus
3 Anconeus
4 Extensor carpi radialis brevis
5 Extensor digitorum
6 Extensor carpi ulnaris
7 Extensor digiti minimi
8 Abductor pollicis longus
9 Extensor pollicis brevis
10 Extensor pollicis longus
11 Ulnar nerve
12 Flexor carpi ulnaris

7.34
Posterior aspect of the elbow and forearm: deep muscles
1 Supinator
2 Abductor pollicis longus
3 Extensor pollicis brevis
4 Extensor pollicis longus
5 Extensor carpi radialis longus
6 Extensor carpi radialis brevis
7 Extensor indicis
8 Flexor carpi ulnaris

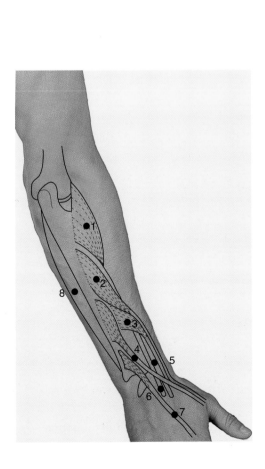

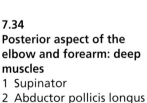

7

MOVEMENTS OF THE ELBOW AND RADIOULNAR JOINTS

The elbow is flexed by the biceps and brachialis muscles, assisted by brachioradialis and the muscles attached to the common flexor origin. Extension is by the triceps muscle, with a weak contribution from the muscles of common extensor origin.

In the anatomical position, the palm faces forwards, the position of the forearm being in full supination (Fig. 7.35). The lower end of the radius may be rotated medially, anterior to the ulna through 180°, to bring the thumb from lateral to medial and the dorsum of the hand anteriorly; this is the position of full pronation (Fig. 7.36). These, and intermediate positions, place the hand in the most appropriate position for a required movement. The biceps and supinator muscles supinate and the pronator teres and pronator quadratus pronate. This last muscle is a deep small muscle joining the anterior aspect of the distal quarter of the radius and ulna near the wrist. The brachioradialis brings the forearm into the midprone position.

In the anatomical position, the styloid processes of the radius and ulna are palpable on their respective sides of the wrist joint; the radial styloid is 1 cm distal to the ulna. In full pronation, the radial styloid is still palpable but medially placed. The bone most easily palpable on the anterolateral aspect of the wrist is now the head of the ulna. The distal end of the ulna undergoes some medial-to-lateral displacement during pronation, this being more marked when the elbow is flexed. However, there is no rotation of the ulna and the styloid process is no longer palpable.

The bone across the supracondylar region of the humerus is very thin in children, and prone to fracture. The distal fragment in this injury is displaced posteriorly and a knuckle of brachial artery may be trapped between the broken bone ends. Radial artery pulsation must be carefully monitored as, if an occluded brachial artery is left untreated, forearm muscle ischaemia can give rise to a contracture (Volkmann's), with long-term disability.

Forearm fractures in children characteristically break along one side of the bone, which bends rather than snaps. This is like a broken sapling branch of a tree, and is thus called a greenstick fracture. In old age, the bones become soft and crumble more easily. A characteristic upper limb fracture in the elderly is through the distal end of the radius, a centimetre proximal to its articular surface (Colles' fracture), sustained by a fall onto the outstretched hand.

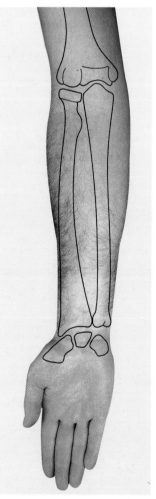

7.35
Forearm in full supination

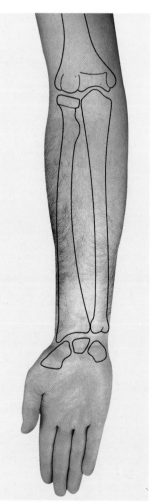

7.36
Forearm in full pronation

ANTERIOR ASPECT OF THE WRIST AND HAND

The bones of the hand and their relation to observable skin creases are shown in Figure 7.38. When flexing the wrist against resistance, three tendons (flexor carpi radialis, palmaris longus and flexor carpi ulnaris) stand out. The radial artery is easily palpable on the lower end of the radius lateral to flexor carpi radialis. This is the usual site to assess the pulse when examining a patient and to establish the rate, rhythm, volume and character of the cardiac output and firmness of the arterial wall. A needle may be inserted into the artery at this point. The flexor carpi radialis is attached distally to the base of the second and third metacarpal bones. The median nerve lies deep to the palmaris longus, which provides some protection to it in cuts across the wrist. The muscle is attached to the flexor retinaculum and the apex of the palmar aponeurosis; it is occasionally absent. The flexor carpi ulnaris muscle is attached to the pisiform bone and thence onto the hamate and the base of the fifth metacarpal bones (Fig. 7.41). The ulnar artery and nerve lie lateral to the tendon but are partly covered by the palmaris brevis muscle and the medial superficial part of the flexor retiniculum; they are not easily palpable.

The flexor retinaculum is a 2.5–3 cm rectangular fibrous band between the pisiform and the hook of the hamate medially and the tubercle of the scaphoid and ridge of the trapezium laterally (Fig. 7.42). The pisiform is easily palpable and the other three bones are felt by deeper palpation. The tendons of the flexor digitorum superficialis and profundus and the flexor pollicis longus are deeply placed anterior to the wrist joint and pass with the median nerve deep to the flexor retinaculum.

The tunnel formed by the retinaculum and the carpus has limited space and an increase in pressure can compress the median nerve, producing pain and numbness in the lateral aspect of the hand, and wasting of the thenar muscles (the carpal tunnel syndrome). The flexor retinaculum may be divided through an incision across the wrist joint to relieve pressure in this condition.

The deep flexor tendons are enclosed in synovial sheaths over the wrist and into the fingers as shown in Figure 7.43. These have clinical significance as infection can spread along a sheath.

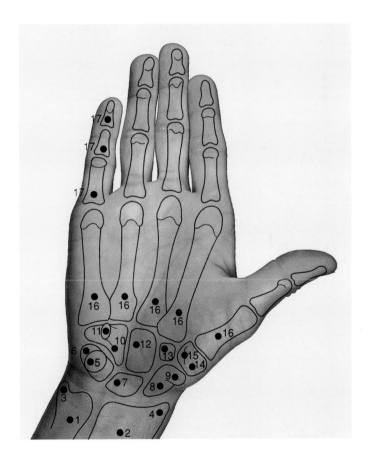

7.38
Anterior aspect of the wrist and hand: bones
Note the relation of bones to the skin creases

1 Ulna	10 Hamate
2 Radius	11 Hook of hamate
3 Ulnar styloid process	12 Capitate
4 Radial styloid process	13 Trapezoid
5 Pisiform	14 Trapezium
6 Triquetral	15 Ridge of trapezium
7 Lunate	16 Metacarpals 1–5
8 Scaphoid	17 Phalanges
9 Scaphoid tubercle	

7.37
Anterior aspect of the wrist and hand

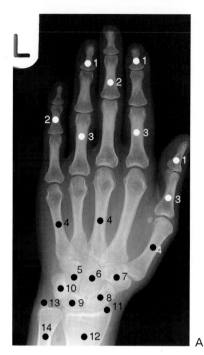

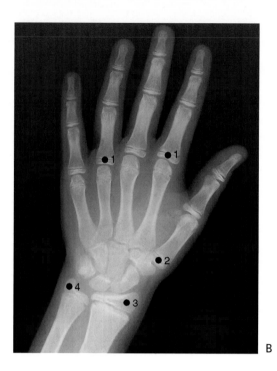

A

B

C

7.39
Wrist joint and hand

A, anterior
1 Terminal phalanx
2 Middle phalanges
3 Proximal phalanges
4 Metacarpals
5 Hamate
6 Capitate
7 Overlapping trapezoid and trapezium
8 Scaphoid

9 Lunate
10 Triquetral, overlapped by pisiform
11 Styloid process of radius
12 Shaft of radius
13 Styloid process of ulna
14 Shaft of ulna

B, anterior view showing epiphyses
1 Epiphysis of proximal phalanx

2 Epiphysis of metacarpal
3 Distal epiphysis of radius
4 Distal epiphysis of ulna

C, lateral view
1 First metacarpal
2 Lunate
3 Overlapping shafts of ulna and radius

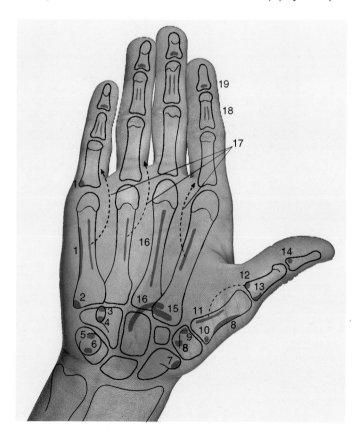

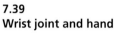

The deep fascia over the palm is thickened centrally to form the palmar aponeurosis which renders the long flexor tendons impalpable at this site. The flexor retinaculum and attachment of the sheaths prevent bowing of the tendons across the wrist during flexion.

The flexor digitorum superficialis and profundus tendons are surrounded by synovial and fibrous sheaths in the fingers and although movement can be felt, individual tendons cannot be palpated. The flexor digitorum profundus is attached to the base of the distal phalanx and the flexor digitorum superficialis tendon divides into two slips which pass on either side of the profundus tendon to be attached to the middle phalanx. The flexor pollicis longus tendon has its own synovial and fibrous sheaths and is attached to the distal phalanx of the thumb.

7.40
Anterior aspect of the wrist and hand: muscle attachments

1 and 3 Opponens digiti minimi
2 Pisometacarpal ligament
4 Flexor digiti minimi
5 Abductor digiti minimi
6 Flexor carpi ulnaris
7 Abductor pollicis brevis
8 Opponens pollicis
9 Flexor pollicis brevis

10 Abductor pollicis longus
11 and 17 Palmar interossei
12 and 16 Adductor pollicis
13 Flexor pollicis brevis and abductor pollicis longus
14 Flexor pollicis longus
15 Flexor carpi radialis
18 Flexor digitorum sublimus
19 Flexor digitorum profundus

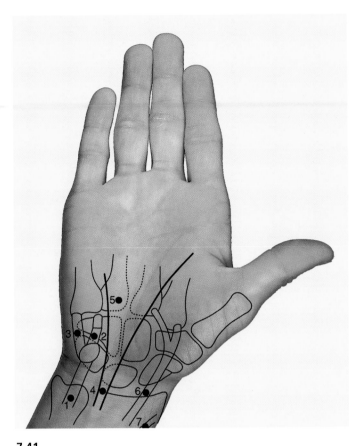

7.41
Anterior aspect of the wrist and hand: superficial tendons

1 Flexor carpi ulnaris
2 Pisohamate ligament
3 Pisometacarpal ligament
4 Palmaris longus
5 Palmar aponeurosis
6 Flexor carpi radialis
7 Radial artery

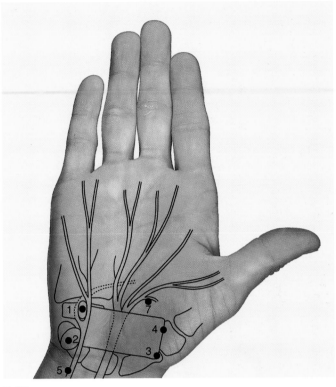

7.42
Flexor retinaculum

1 Hook of hamate
2 Pisiform bone
3 Scaphoid tubercle
4 Ridge of trapezium
5 Ulnar nerve
6 Median nerve
7 Recurrent branch of
   median nerve

The skin of the palm is hairless and thickened. The configuration of dermal papillae serves to anchor the epidermis to the dermis, providing a friction surface for gripping and other manual tasks; fibrofatty compartments over the palm produce a firm cushioned area of contact. The palm has a large number of sweat glands which serve to cool the surface during activity and maintain the suppleness of the skin.

The skin over the dorsum of the hand is more mobile and elastic than that of the palm, allowing for stretching during full finger and wrist flexion. The hand, particularly at the fingertips, is densely innervated, these sensory nerve endings facilitating delicate tactile discrimination, such as in reading Braille and feeling in the dark and around corners.

The nail is attached to the surrounding skin by the cuticle (eponychium). Infection may enter a break in this layer, resulting in inflammation of the surrounding tissues and the formation of pus under the nail, a condition known as a paronychia.

7.43
Anterior aspect of the wrist and hand: digital flexor tendons and sheaths

1 Flexor digitorum superficialis
2 Flexor digitorum profundus
3 Flexor pollicis longus

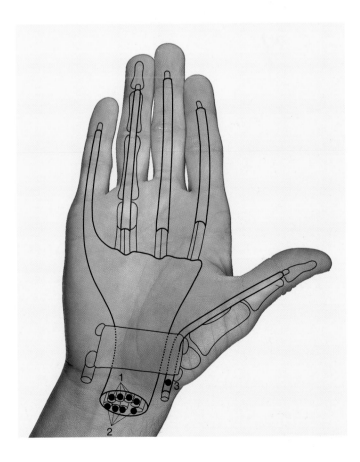

ANATOMICAL SNUFF BOX

The anatomical snuff box is a depression on the lateral aspect of the wrist which is accentuated when the thumb is extended. The bones of its floor are the radial styloid, the wrist joint, the scaphoid, trapezium and the base of the first metacarpal (Fig. 7.45).

Tenderness at this site occurs with injuries of the scaphoid bone and synovitis of the adjacent tendon sheaths.

The snuff box is bounded anteriorly by the tendons of abductor pollicis longus and extensor pollicis brevis and posteriorly by extensor pollicis longus (Fig. 7.46). These three muscles are deeply placed in the forearm and are supplied by the posterior interosseous nerve.

The abductor pollicis longus is attached distally to the first metacarpal and the extensor pollicis brevis to the proximal phalanx of the thumb. The extensor pollicis longus is attached to the distal phalanx of the thumb. The fossa is crossed by the tendons

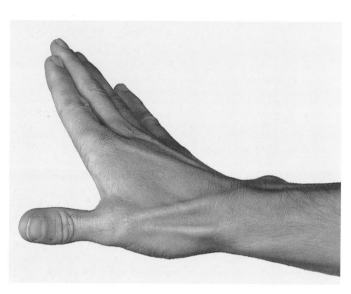

7.44
Anatomical snuff box

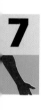

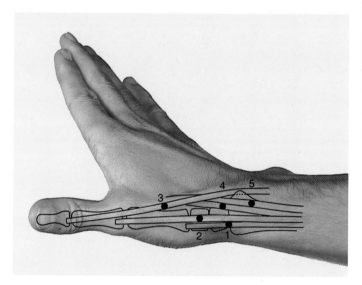

7.46
Anatomical snuff box: tendons
1 Abductor pollicis longus
2 Extensor pollicis brevis
3 Extensor pollicis longus
4 Extensor carpi radialis longus
5 Extensor carpi radialis brevis

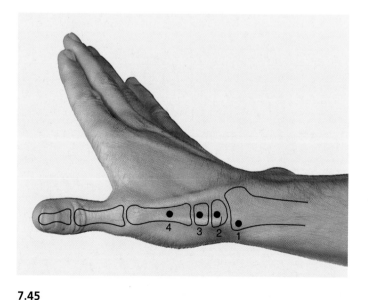

7.45
Anatomical snuff box: bones
1 Radial styloid
2 Scaphoid
3 Trapezium
4 First metacarpal

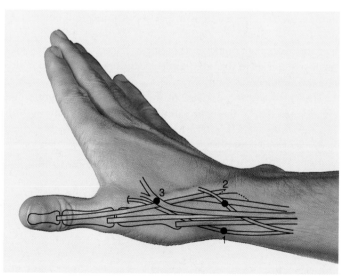

7.47
Anatomical snuff box: radial artery and nerve, and cephalic vein
1 Radial artery
2 Radial nerve
3 Cephalic vein

of the extensor carpi radialis longus and brevis as these pass, respectively, to the bases of the second and third metacarpals. Dorsal digital branches of the radial nerve cross the extensor pollicis longus tendon, just proximal to the snuff box, and are palpable (Fig. 7.47). The radial artery crosses the lateral aspect of the wrist before passing between the first and second metacarpals into the palm. Its pulsation can be felt in the floor of the snuff box. The cephalic vein crosses the fossa superficially.

DORSAL ASPECT OF THE WRIST AND HAND

The distal end of the radius is palpable posteriorly, particularly the dorsal tubercle, around which hooks the tendon of extensor pollicis longus. The triquetral, lunate and scaphoid bones, from medial to lateral, form the distal articulation of the wrist joint (Fig. 7.49). These, other carpal bones and the bases of the medial four metacarpals are not easily palpated. The remainder of the metacarpals and phalanges can be palpated throughout their length posteriorly. A finger placed in the depression over the middle of the wrist joint lies between the radius proximally, while distally the finger is related to the capitate on full extension and the lunate on full flexion. The second to fourth metacarpophalangeal joints are easily palpable posteriorly. The first metacarpal is far more mobile than the second to fourth and its carpometacarpal joint is readily palpable. The interphalangeal joints are palpable around their circumference.

The digital extensor tendons are closely related to the posterior aspect of the radius and retain their relations during pronation. They are held down to the bone by a fibrous sheet, the extensor retinaculum. This passes obliquely from the lateral side of the distal radius to the medial side of the carpus; septa from it pass between the extensor tendons forming osseofascial tunnels

(Fig. 7.51). Synovial sheaths cover the tendons beneath and distal to the retinaculum. Each extensor digitorum tendon forms a triangle (the dorsal expansion) over the metacarpophalangeal joint. The corresponding interossei and lumbrical muscles are attached to the base of this expansion. At the apex of the triangle the long tendon reforms and then divides into three slips over the proximal interphalangeal joint. The middle slip is attached to the base of the middle phalanx and the outer slips reunite before being attached to the base of the terminal phalanx.

Two further tendons may be visible on the dorsum of the wrist. The extensor digiti minimi lies medial to the long tendon of the little finger and is inserted into its dorsal tendinous expansion. The extensor indicis is a deep muscle of the forearm supplied by the posterior interosseous nerve; its tendon lies medial to the long tendon of the index finger and it is also inserted into the dorsal expansion. Both extensor digiti minimi and extensor indicis tendons can be removed and used for grafting

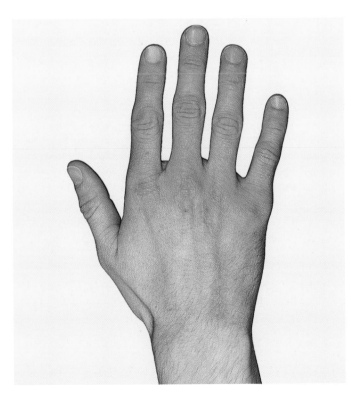

7.48
Dorsal aspect of the supine wrist and hand

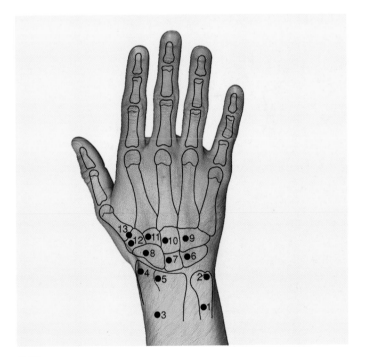

7.49
Dorsal aspect of the wrist and hand: bones

1 Ulna	8 Scaphoid
2 Ulna styloid	9 Hamate
3 Radius	10 Capitate
4 Radial styloid	11 Trapezoid
5 Dorsal tubercle of radius	12 Trapezium
6 Triquetral	13 Carpometacarpal joint
7 Lunate	of thumb

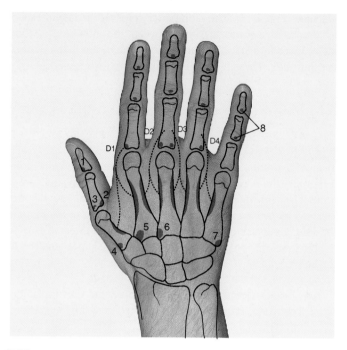

7.50
Dorsal aspect of the wrist and hand: muscle attachments

1 Extensor pollicis longus
2 Adductor pollicis
3 Extensor pollicis brevis
4 Abductor pollicis longus
5 Extensor carpi radialis longus

6 Extensor carpi radialis brevis
7 Extensor carpi ulnaris
8 Extensor digitorum

D1–4 dorsal interossei

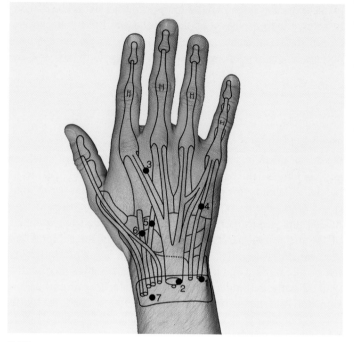

7.51
Dorsal aspect of the wrist and hand: tendons

1 Extensor carpi ulnaris
2 Extensor digitorum
3 Extensor indicis
4 Extensor digiti minimi
5 Extensor carpi radialis brevis

6 Extensor carpi radialis longus
7 Extensor retinaculum

with minimal loss of function in the hand. The veins over the dorsum of the hand are usually prominent and provide useful sites for venous access, as does the cephalic vein over the anatomical snuff box.

Note that Figures 7.45–7.47 are with the forearm and hand in pronation with the head of the ulna prominent. In contrast, Figures 7.48–7.51 are with the forearm and hand in supination and the styloid process of the ulna can be seen.

MOVEMENTS OF THE WRIST AND HAND

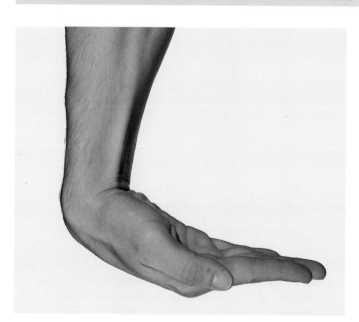

Movements at the wrist (radiocarpal) joint are combined with and augmented by movement at the midcarpal (between the proximal and distal rows of the carpus) joint. Flexion occurs mainly at the midcarpal joint and is produced by the flexor carpi radialis and flexor carpi ulnaris assisted by the long digital flexor muscles (Fig. 7.52). Extension is mainly at the wrist joint and is produced by the extensor carpi radialis longus and brevis and the extensor carpi ulnaris, assisted by the long digital extensor muscles (Fig. 7.53). Abduction is mainly at the midcarpal joint and produced by flexor carpi radialis and extensor carpi radialis longus and brevis (Fig. 7.54). Adduction is mainly at the wrist joint and produced by the flexor carpi ulnaris and extensor carpi ulnaris (Fig. 7.55).

7.52
Wrist flexion

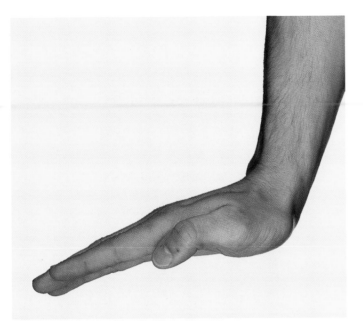

7.53
Wrist extension

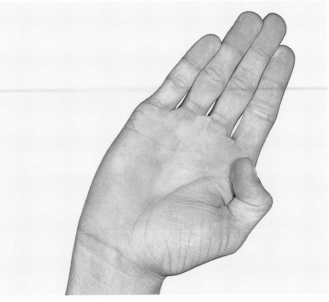

7.54
Wrist abduction

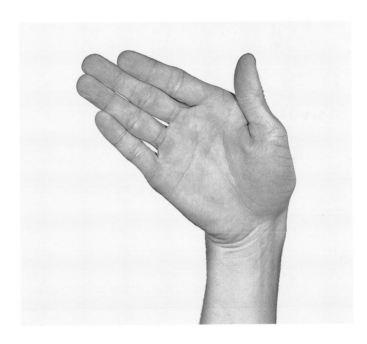

7.55
Wrist adduction

7

THENAR AND HYPOTHENAR EMINENCES

Thenar eminence

The muscle bulk of the lateral aspect of the palm is known as the thenar eminence and it is formed by the short muscles of the thumb. The abductor, flexor and opponens pollicis muscles are attached to the scaphoid tubercle, the ridge of the trapezium and the adjacent flexor retinaculum. The abductor pollicis brevis and flexor pollicis brevis also pass to the radial side of the proximal phalanx of the thumb and the opponens pollicis to the whole length of the radial margin of the first metacarpal bone. The three muscles are supplied by the median nerve, by a recurrent branch after the nerve exits from the carpal tunnel. The adductor

pollicis is deeply placed in the palm and is attached medially by two heads to the capitate and second and third metacarpals and laterally to the proximal phalanx of the thumb. It is supplied by the ulnar nerve. The muscle bulk in the first intermetacarpal space includes adductor pollicis, the first dorsal and palmar interossei, and the first lumbrical.

There is considerable mobility at the saddle-shaped carpo-metacarpal joint of the thumb. Movements are described in relation to the plane of the nail bed rather than the coronal plane of the body. Flexion is combined with medial rotation and is produced by flexor pollicis longus and brevis and opponens

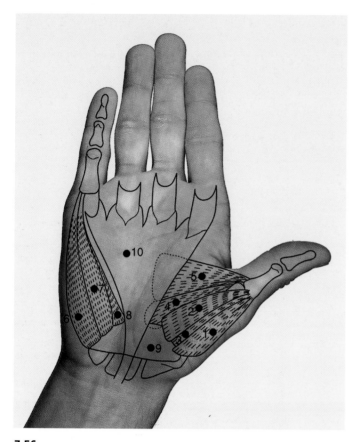

7.56
Thenar and hypothenar eminences

1 Abductor pollicis brevis	6 Abductor digiti minimi
2 Flexor pollicis brevis	7 Flexor digiti minimi
3 Opponens pollicis	8 Opponens digiti minimi
4 Adductor pollicis oblique head	9 Flexor retinaculum
5 Adductor pollicis transverse head	10 Palmar aponeurosis

pollicis. Extension is combined with lateral rotation and brought about by extensor pollicis longus and brevis and abductor pollicis longus. The abductor pollicis brevis produces abduction (away from the palm, in the plane of the nail, i.e. 90° to the plane of the palm), the adductor pollicis adduction (return from the abducted position), and the opponens pollicis opposition to the index and other digits.

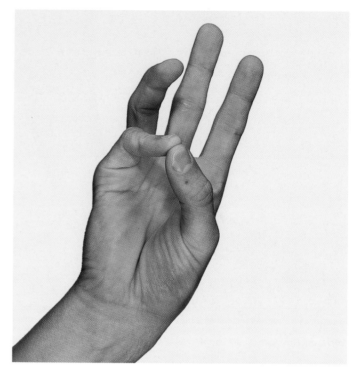

7.57
Flexion and opposition of the thumb and little finger
(Movement: 2/3 thumb, 1/3 little finger)

Hypothenar eminence

The hypothenar eminence is formed by the abductor digiti minimi, flexor digiti minimi and opponens digiti minimi, arising from the flexor retinaculum and adjacent medial bones, and passing distally to the ulnar side of the proximal phalanx and the ulnar margin of the fifth metacarpal bone. The little finger is less mobile than the thumb, but slight rotation is present. The muscles are supplied by the ulnar nerve. The thenar and hypothenar muscles are within their own osseofascial compartment of deep fascia.

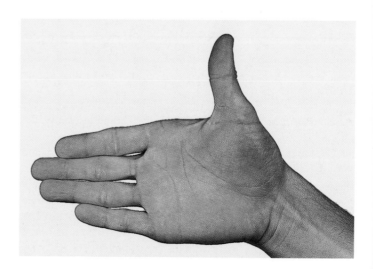

7.58
Extension of the thumb

Interosseous muscles

Movements of the carpometacarpal joint of the thumb and all metacarpophalangeal joints are flexion, extension, abduction, adduction, circumduction and some rotation. For digits 2–5 (index to minimus), flexion and extension are in the sagittal plane, while abduction and adduction are in the coronal plane (i.e. the plane of the palm). Movements of the thumb are at 90° to the other digits, flexion and extension in the coronal plane (i.e. the plane of the palm), abduction and adduction in the sagittal plane; a combination of abduction, flexion and medial rotation produces opposition of the thumb. In Figure 7.57, the minimus is flexed and laterally rotated in opposition to the thumb. Abduction and adduction of digits 2–5 (away from and towards the midline of the middle finger) are brought about by the palmar and dorsal interosseous muscles arising from the sides of the length of the metacarpals and forming the muscle bulk palpable between these bones; this is particularly marked between the first and second metacarpals. The four smaller palmar interosseous muscles are attached to the palmar surfaces of the first, second, fourth and fifth metacarpal bones.

The four dorsal interosseous muscles are larger and more powerful, arising by two heads from the adjacent sides of the metacarpal bones. The distal tendons of all the interossei gain attachment to the corresponding proximal phalanx and extensor expansion. These attachments are such that the palmar muscles adduct (PAD) and the dorsal muscles abduct (DAB). The interossei also flex the proximal phalanx at the metacarpophalangeal

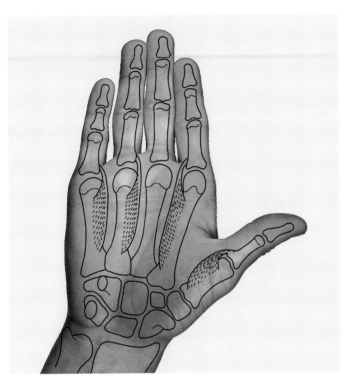

7.59
Palmar interossei

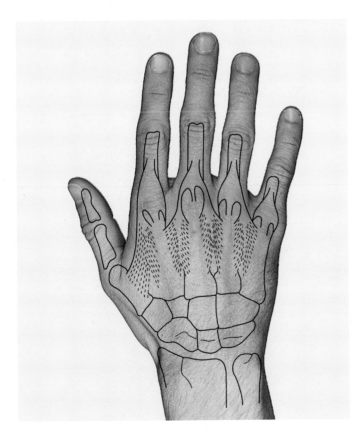

7.60
Dorsal interossei

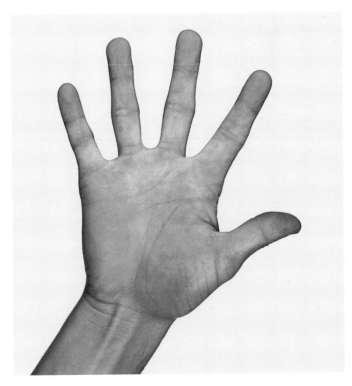

7.61
Finger abduction and extension with thumb extension

7

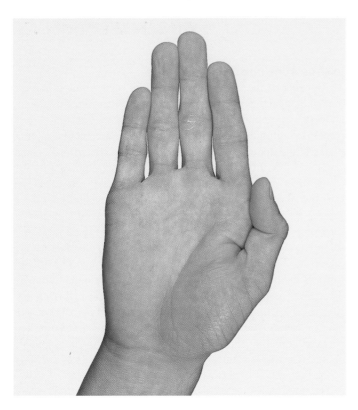

7.62
Finger adduction and extension
Thumb in adducted position: note partial flexion of its
metacarpophalangeal and solitary interphalangeal joints

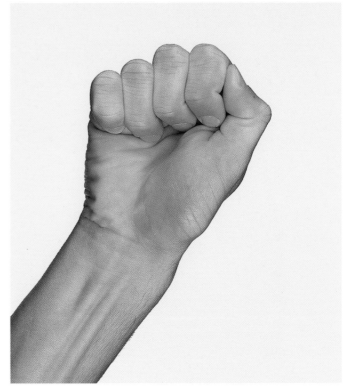

7.63
Finger flexion

Extension of the fingers is mainly by the long digital extensor muscles aided by extensor indicis and extensor digiti minimi. The collateral slips of the extensor expansion over the proximal interphalangeal joint reunite beyond the expansion. The reformed tendon is attached to the base of the distal phalanx and extends the distal interphalangeal joint.

joint and, through their attachment to the extensor expansion, extend the proximal and distal interphalangeal joints.

Lumbrical muscles

The lumbricals are four slender muscles arising from the lateral side of each flexor digitorum profundus tendon in the palm; they are attached to the lateral side of the dorsal expansion of the same finger. Their action is to flex the metacarpophalangeal joint and extend the proximal and distal interphalangeal joints, aided by the interosseous muscles.

All the interosseous and the medial two lumbrical muscles are supplied by the ulnar nerve and the lateral two lumbricals by the median nerve. Further flexion of the metacarpal and interphalangeal joints of the finger is by the long flexor tendons; the flexor digitorum profundus alone acts on the distal interphalangeal joint.

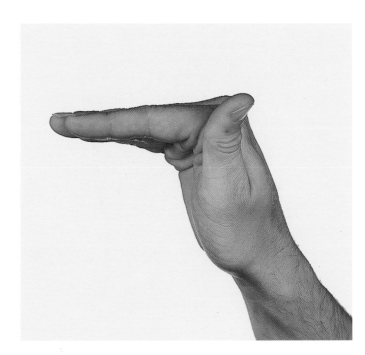

7.64
Action of the lumbrical muscles

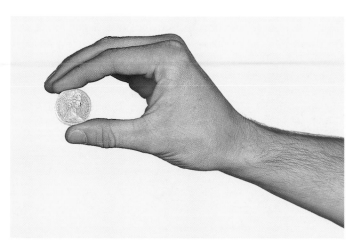

7.65
Precision grip

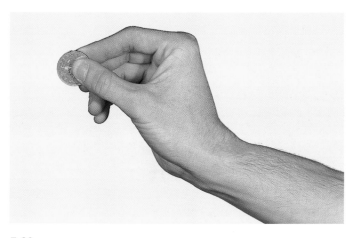

7.66
Pinch grip

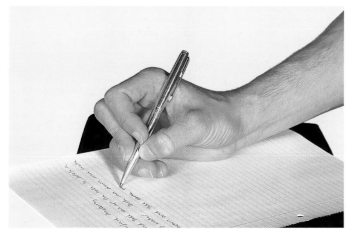

7.67
Writing

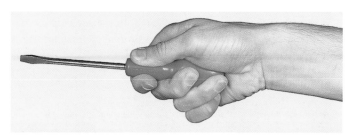

7.68
Power grip

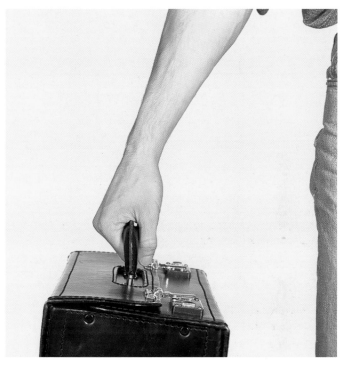

7.69
Hook grip

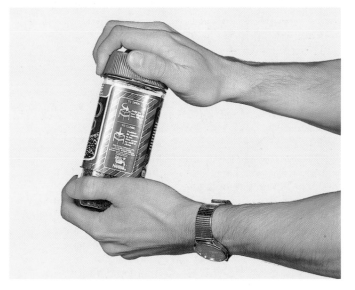

7.70
Unscrewing the top of a jar

7

INNERVATION OF THE UPPER LIMB

The innervation of a limb (arm or leg) follows three distinctive patterns of clinical relevance in terms of their segmental origin and distribution. They reflect their different modes of development: these are (a) cutaneous, (b) to the muscles and joints, and (c) autonomic. Relevant terms are: axis of the limb; preaxial border (lateral border, radial border, bearing the thumb and cephalic vein); postaxial border (medial border, ulnar border, bearing the little finger and basilic vein); apex of the limb (middle three digits); dermatome (skin area supplied by a single spinal nerve) and myotome (muscle volume supplied by a single spinal nerve).

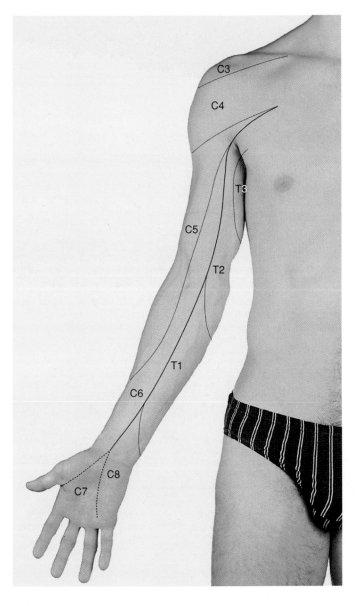

7.71
Cutaneous nerves of the upper limb: anterior

1 Supraclavicular
2 Upper lateral cutaneous nerve of arm
3 Intercostobrachial
4 Anterior cutaneous nerve of arm (branch of 5)
5 Medial cutaneous nerve of arm
6 Medial cutaneous nerve of forearm
7 Lateral cutaneous nerve of forearm
8 Palmar branch of ulnar
9 Palmar branch of median
10 Superficial terminal branch of radial
11 Ulnar digital
12 Median digital

7.72
Cutaneous dermatomes of the upper limb: anterior
The numbers denote the nerve roots. The dark line is the anterior axial line
C, cervical; T, thoracic

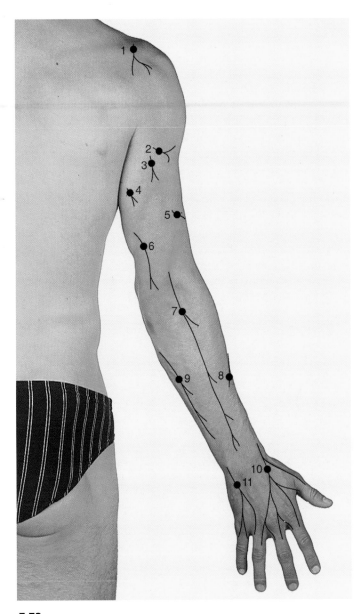

7.73
Cutaneous nerves of the upper limb: posterior

1 Supraclavicular
2 Upper lateral cutaneous nerve of arm
3 Posterior cutaneous nerve of arm
4 Intercostobrachial
5 Lower lateral cutaneous nerve of arm
6 Medial cutaneous nerve of arm
7 Posterior cutaneous nerve of forearm
8 Lateral cutaneous nerve of forearm
9 Medial cutaneous nerve of forearm
10 Radial
11 Dorsal branch of ulnar

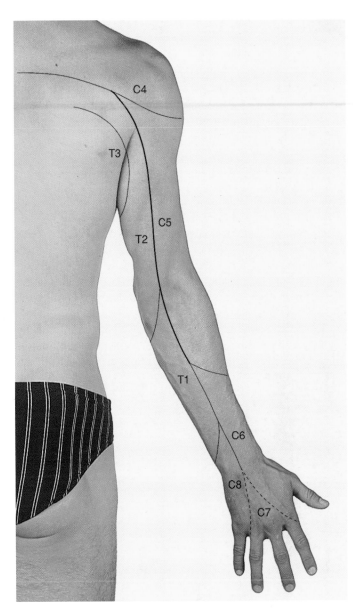

7.74
Cutaneous dermatomes of the upper limb: posterior
The numbers denote the nerve roots. The dark line is the posterior axial line
C, cervical; T, thoracic

The highest (spinal nerve level) dermatome is at the preaxial root of the limb, then successive dermatomes proceed down the preaxial border to the apex, and then return along the postaxial border to reach the trunk at the limb root. Areas supplied by successive dermatomes have considerable overlap in their innervation. Areas supplied by discontinuous (non-successive dermatomes) have minimal or no overlap; these are the dorsal and ventral axial lines (Figs 7.72, 7.74).

In contrast, the highest myotomes (spinal nerve level) are sited proximally, the intermediate where their name implies, and the lowest are distal (the intrinsic muscles of the hand or foot).

The skin of the upper limb is supplied by the C5 to T1 dermatomes but with additions from C4 and T2, 3 through the brachial plexus. The fourth cervical root supplies the skin over the tip of the shoulder and the third thoracic that over the axilla. The sixth root supplies the skin over the thumb and the eighth that of the little finger. The distribution of the seventh root to the central fingers is variable. When testing for sensory disturbance,

7

the greatest difference can be demonstrated across axial lines because of the considerable overlap between the innervation of adjacent dermatomes elsewhere.

In brachial plexus injuries of the upper trunk (C5, 6 – birth injuries and severe downward traction on the shoulder), the deltoid, teres minor, supraspinatus, infraspinatus, biceps and brachialis and sometimes other muscles are paralysed. The limb hangs limply, medially rotated and fully pronated, in the 'tip' position. There is sensory diminution on the radial side of the arm and forearm. Lower trunk injuries (C8, T1) can also occur at birth, from grasping overhead to break a fall or from pressure from a cervical rib; they produce paralysis of the small muscles of the hand and the long digital flexors, resulting in the characteristic clawed hand, and sensory diminution on the ulnar side of the arm and forearm.

Axillary nerve injuries are usually associated with dislocation of the shoulder joint or during its reduction, and fractures of the surgical neck of the humerus; they result in paralysis of the deltoid muscle and anaesthesia of the skin over the deltoid tuberosity. The radial nerve is most easily damaged in fractures of the humerus as it crosses the radial groove. As the triceps muscle is supplied from above this level, the disability is paralysis of the wrist extensor muscles (wrist drop). Sensory loss is distal to the snuff box and often minimal.

Median nerve injuries are commonest in the carpal tunnel, resulting in paralysis of the thenar muscles (except adductor pollicis) and the lateral two lumbricals. There is sensory palmar loss over the thumb, index, middle and half the ring finger. More proximal injuries result in additional paralysis of the forearm flexors and absence of pronation.

The ulnar nerve is subject to injury as it crosses the posterior aspect of the medial epicondyle of the humerus. There is paralysis of all the remaining small muscles of the hand, and also flexor carpi ulnaris and part of flexor digitorum profundus; sensory loss is over the ulnar side of the hand. When the long digital flexor muscles can contract unopposed by lumbricals and interossei, as with injuries of the ulnar or median nerves at the wrist, there is clawing of the hand.

The biceps reflex is lost with lesions of the fifth and sixth roots, the brachioradialis with the sixth, and the triceps with the sixth and seventh cervical root injuries.

The preganglionic autonomic supply to the arm is from T2 to T6.

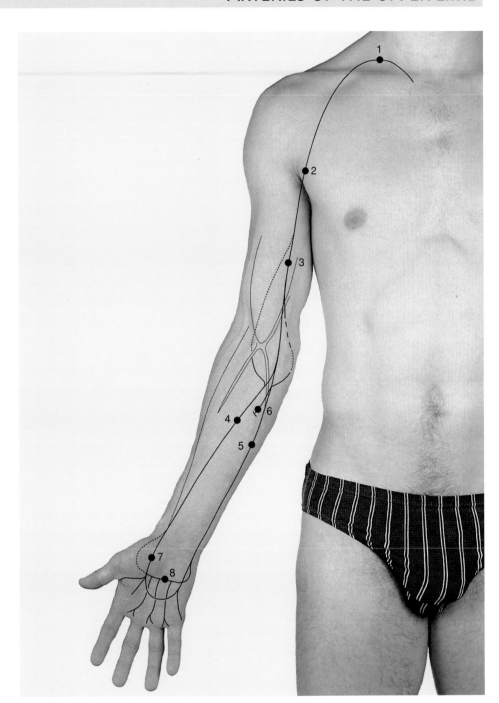

7.75
Arteries of the upper limb
1 Subclavian
2 Axillary
3 Brachial
4 Radial
5 Ulnar
6 Common interosseous
7 Superficial palmar arch
8 Deep palmar arch

7

8 LOWER LIMB

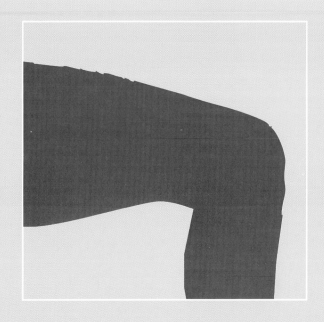

FEMORAL TRIANGLE

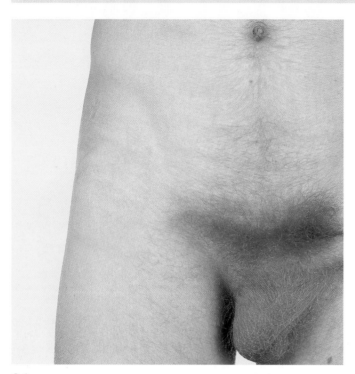

8.1
Femoral triangle

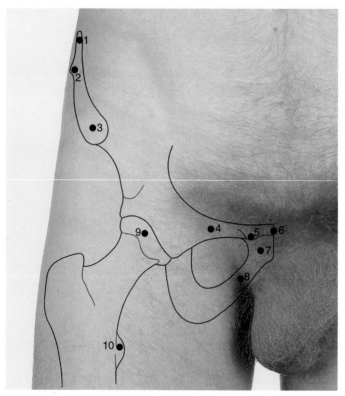

8.2
Femoral triangle: bones

1	Iliac crest	6	Symphysis pubis
2	Iliac tubercle	7	Body of pubis
3	Anterior superior iliac spine	8	Inferior pubic ramus
4	Superior pubic ramus	9	Head of femur
5	Pubic tubercle	10	Lesser trochanter

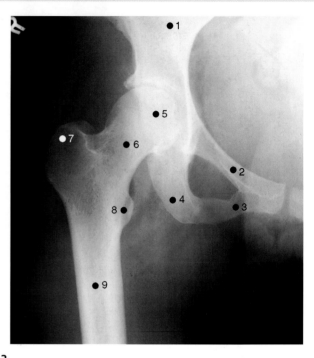

8.3
Hip and pelvis: anterior view

1	Ilium	6	Neck of femur
2	Superior ramus of pubis	7	Greater trochanter
3	Inferior ramus of pubis	8	Lesser trochanter
4	Ischium	9	Shaft of femur
5	Head of femur		

The symphysis, body, crest and tubercle of the pubis, and the anterior superior iliac spine of the pelvis are palpable anteriorly (Fig. 8.2). The inguinal ligament passes between the anterior superior iliac spine and the pubic tubercle, and forms about three-quarters of the base of the femoral triangle (the rest continues across the body of the pubis – Figs 8.5, 8.7). The lateral border of the triangle is formed by the sartorius muscle. This muscle passes from the anterior superior iliac spine distally, across the thigh, to be attached to the medial subcutaneous surface of the upper tibia. Its function is best described as producing the crossed-leg position and it is known as the tailor's muscle; it is supplied by the femoral nerve.

The medial border of the triangle is the medial aspect of the adductor longus muscle passing from the body of the pubis to the linea aspera of the femur; it is supplied by the obturator nerve. The roof of the triangle is formed of fascia lata, which surrounds the thigh like a stocking and is attached superiorly to the inguinal ligament, the iliac crest, the inferior pubic ramus and the sacrum. The saphenous opening in the fascia is 4 cm below and just lateral to the pubic tubercle, overlying the femoral vein and transmitting its great saphenous tributary.

The floor of the triangle is formed by the iliopsoas and pectineus muscles which lie anterior to the hip joint; the head of the femur can be felt deeply in the triangle. The iliopsoas muscle is attached proximally to the medial aspect of the ilium and to the lateral aspect of the lumbar vertebrae. Distally, the tendon passes to the lesser trochanter of the femur; it is a powerful flexor and

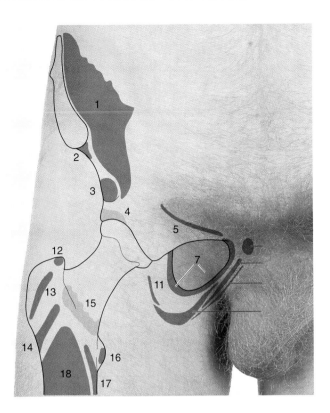

8.4
Femoral triangle: muscle attachments

1 Iliacus	8 Adductor brevis
2 Sartorius	9 Gracilis
3 Rectus femoris	10 Adductor longus
4 and 15 Iliofemoral	11 Quadratus femoris
ligament	12 Piriformis
5 Pectineus	13 Gluteus maximus
6 Adductor longus	14 Vastus lateralis
7 Obturator externus (from	16 Psoas major
ischium and obturator	17 Vastus medialis
membrane)	18 Vastus intermedius

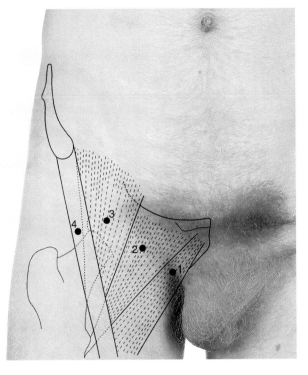

8.5
Femoral triangle: muscles

1 Adductor longus	3 Iliopsoas
2 Pectineus	4 Sartorius

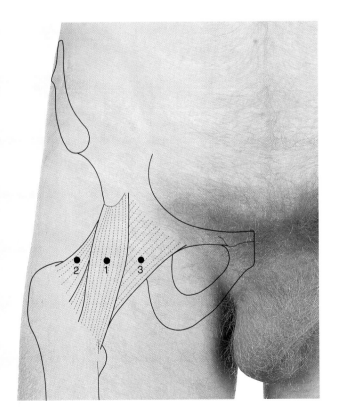

8.6
Hip joint: anterior aspect
1 and 2 Iliofemoral ligament
3 Pubofemoral ligament

medial rotator of the hip joint and is supplied from the lumbar plexus through the second and third roots. The pectineus muscle is attached to the superior pubic ramus and, distally, just below the iliopsoas tendon on the femur, it is supplied by the femoral nerve.

The femoral artery descends vertically through the triangle from the midinguinal point (midway between the anterior superior iliac spine and the symphysis pubis) to the apex of the triangle. Its deep (profunda) branch passes posteriorly, between the adductor longus and the pectineus muscles.

The femoral vein lies medial to the artery within a common sheath and with the femoral canal further medially. The femoral nerve lies lateral to the artery, outside the femoral sheath.

The femoral artery is an important site for vascular access and a large number of arteriographic procedures are undertaken through its percutaneous puncture. The femoral vein is also a useful site for venous sampling when other superficial veins, such as those over the cubital fossa, are ill-defined. The femoral artery is prone to arterial disease and the vessel is approached

8

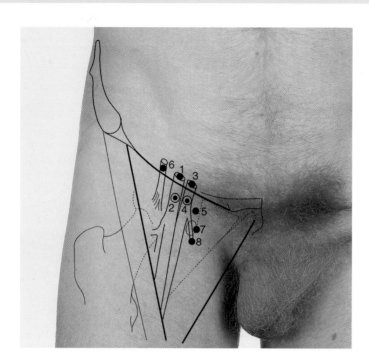

for surgical procedures through a longitudinal incision over the vessel in the femoral triangle.

The inguinal region is examined routinely for lymph node enlargement. Inguinal lymph nodes may be enlarged as part of a generalised disease or secondary to disease of the lower limb. Upper and lower superficial inguinal groups are situated below and parallel to the inguinal ligament, and around the terminal few centimetres of the great saphenous vein, respectively. They drain to the deep inguinal lymph nodes in the femoral canal and thence to the external iliac nodes. Maldevelopment of the lower limb lymphatics may give rise to inadequate drainage of the limb; the swelling produced is termed lymphoedema.

8.7
Femoral triangle: vessels and nerves

1 Femoral artery
2 Point of access to femoral artery
3 Femoral vein
4 Point of access to femoral vein
5 Femoral canal
6 Femoral nerve
7 Saphenous opening
8 Great saphenous vein

ANTERIOR AND MEDIAL ASPECT OF THE HIP, THIGH AND KNEE

Anterior and medial aspect of the thigh

The anterior aspect of the thigh is formed mainly of the large quadriceps muscle mass (Fig. 8.12). The quadriceps has four proximal attachments: the rectus femoris is attached by a straight head to the anterior inferior iliac spine, and by an oblique head to just above the acetabulum. The vastus lateralis and medialis take their attachment from their respective sides of the intertrochanteric line, encircle the subtrochanteric femur, then converge to their respective sides of the linea aspera of the femur and the vastus intermedialis from the anterior aspect of the femoral shaft. The quadriceps muscle is attached inferiorly to the patella and is extended beyond it to form a strong tendon, the patellar 'ligament', attached to the tibial tuberosity. The patella is subcutaneous and easily palpable, as is the tibial tuberosity.

On each side of the patellar ligament, the capsule of the joint is formed largely of downward fibrous expansions of the quadriceps tendon known as retinacula, through which the muscle gains attachment to the tibial condyles. The muscle is supplied by the femoral nerve. The proximal components of the quadriceps are not easily demonstrated when recumbent, or during easy standing, but are clearly seen when the whole leg, with extended knee, is raised against gravity; the patellar ligament and the lower horizontal fibres of the vastus medialis, passing to the medial aspect of the patella, are visible. The latter fibres quickly waste away with inactivity. The medial and lateral femoral condyles and the upper margin of the tibia can be palpated over most of the anterior, medial and lateral aspects of the knee joint. (Fig. 8.9).

The medial side of the thigh contains the adductor group of muscles. The first layer, the pectineus and the adductor longus, has been described in the femoral triangle; the adductor brevis passes from the inferior pubic ramus to the linea aspera between these muscles and the more deeply placed powerful adductor magnus

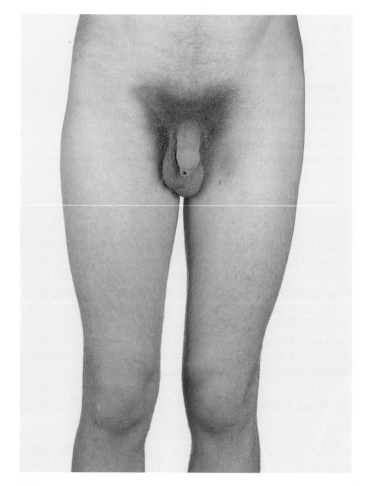

8.8
Anterior and medial aspect of the thigh

(Fig. 8.12). The latter is attached medially along the ischiopubic ramus and ischial tuberosity and, laterally, to the length of the linea aspera and the medial supracondylar ridge and by a strong tendon to the adductor tubercle on the femur. The tubercle is palpable. The femoral vessels pass through a defect (the adductor hiatus) in this asperal attachment close to the femur; at this point they become the popliteal vessels. The opening is approximately 10 cm above the knee joint. The adductor muscles are overlain by the gracilis muscle, a thin flat (gracile) muscle passing from the inferior pubic ramus to the upper medial aspect of the tibia. The gracilis and the adductor muscles adduct the hip joint and are supplied by the obturator nerve. The adductor magnus also has a sciatic nerve supply to that part arising from the ischial tuberosity; this is functionally and developmentally a part of the hamstring muscle group extending the hip joint.

Medial aspect of the knee

The medial collateral ligament of the knee joint is a wide, flat, strong sheet blending with the capsule of the joint, passing from the medial epicondyle of the femur to the upper surface of the tibial shaft (Fig. 8.15, Fig 8.44, p. 110). The medial edge of

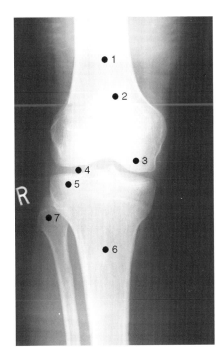

8.10
The knee joint: anterior view
1 Femoral shaft
2 Upper border of patella
3 Medial femoral condyle
4 Joint space of the knee
5 Lateral tibial condyle
6 Tibial shaft
7 Head of fibula

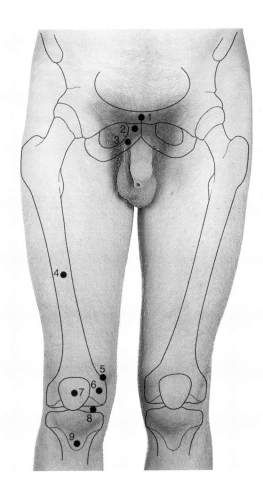

8.9
Anterior and medial aspect of the thigh: bones
1 Symphysis pubis
2 Body of pubis
3 Inferior pubic ramus
4 Femur
5 Adductor tubercle
6 Medial femoral condyle
7 Patella
8 Tibial plateau
9 Tibial tuberosity

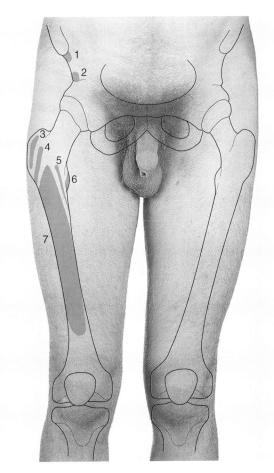

8.11
Anterior and medial aspect of thigh: muscle attachments
1 Sartorius
2 Rectus femoris
3 Gluteus minimus
4 Vastus lateralis
5 Vastus medialis
6 Psoas major
7 Vastus intermedius

8

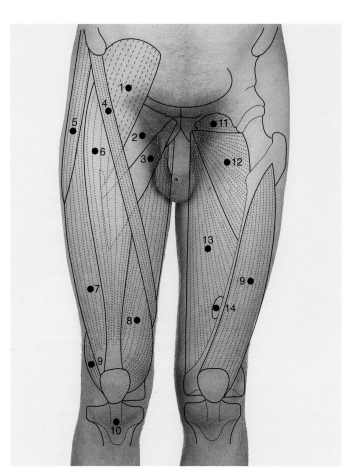

8.12

Anterior and medial aspect of the thigh: superficial (right limb) and deep (left limb) muscles

(Items 6–10 make up the quadriceps muscle)

1	Iliopsoas	8	Vastus medialis
2	Pectineus	9	Vastus intermedius
3	Adductor longus	10	Patellar tendon
4	Sartorius	11	Obturator externus
5	Tensor fascia lata	12	Adductor brevis
6	Rectus femoris	13	Adductor magnus
7	Vastus lateralis	14	Adductor hiatus

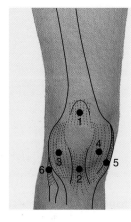

8.13

Knee joint: anterior aspect

1	Tendon of quadriceps	4	Medial patellar retinaculum
2	Ligamentum patellae	5	Medial ligament
3	Lateral patellar retinaculum	6	Lateral ligament

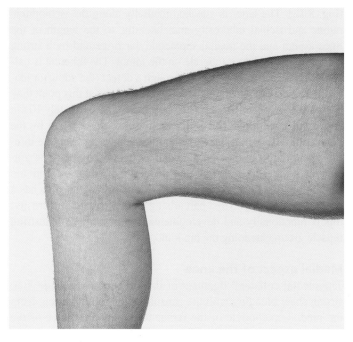

8.14
Medial aspect of the flexed knee

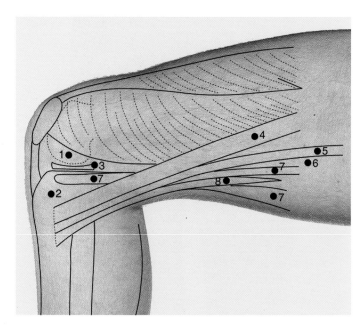

8.15
Medial aspect of the flexed knee: bones and muscles

1	Medial femoral condyle	5	Gracilis
2	Medial tibial condyle	6	Adductor magnus
3	Medial meniscus	7	Semimembranosus
4	Sartorius	8	Semitendinosus

the medial meniscus is between the femoral and tibial condyles; although it is normally impalpable, if damaged, tenderness can be noted along the joint line and there may be a protrusion over the site of a tear. The tendons of the sartorius, gracilis and semi-tendinosus are attached to the subcutaneous upper surface of the tibia, from anterior to posterior; they are more easily defined with the knee flexed to a right angle.

LATERAL ASPECT OF THE HIP, THIGH AND KNEE

Lateral aspect of the hip

The greater trochanter is palpable on the upper lateral aspect of the thigh: it lies posterior and distal to the anterior superior iliac spine.

When sitting, the body weight is taken on the ischial tuberosities and is cushioned by the mass of the gluteus maximus and the fatty tissues of the buttock.

In fractures of the neck of the femur the distance BC in the triangle shown in Figure 8.17 (Bryant's triangle) is shortened and this can be demonstrated by comparing the normal and fractured sides.

Fractures of the neck of the femur are common in the elderly, particularly after a fall and often after seemingly minor trauma. Severe trauma can produce fractures of the femoral shaft and, if directed along the length of the femur, such as in motorcycle accidents, it can produce posterior dislocation of the hip joint. In the latter case, the posterior rim of the acetabulum is usually fractured and the sciatic nerve may be damaged. Knee fractures are usually due to direct trauma. They involve the femoral and tibial condyles, and may traverse the articular surfaces of the joint. Torsion injuries can damage the collateral ligaments and the intra-articular menisci.

Lateral aspect of the knee

The biceps tendon can be clearly defined over the lateral aspect of the knee when the knee is flexed to a right angle; the tendon can be followed to its attachment to the upper end of the fibula (Figs 8.24, 8.49, p. 112). The bony margin of the lateral aspect of the tibial condyle can be palpated and the fibular (lateral collateral) ligament felt as a firm cord, separate from the joint capsule, passing from the lateral aspect of the femoral condyle to the head of the fibula. The lateral meniscus lies adjacent to the tibial margin and becomes tender and sometimes palpable when damaged. The common peroneal nerve is overlapped by the tendon of the biceps and then passes subcutaneously over the neck of the fibula, where it can be palpated, before it divides into deep and superficial branches that enter the anterior and lateral compartments of the leg, respectively.

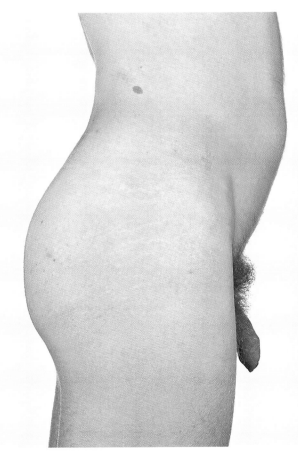

8.16
Lateral aspect of the hip joint

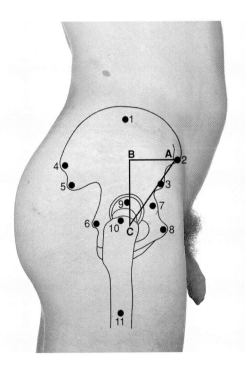

8.17
Lateral aspect of the hip joint: bones

1 Ilium	6 Ischial spine
2 Anterior superior iliac spine	7 Iliopubic eminence
	8 Body of pubis
3 Anterior inferior iliac spine	9 Head of femur
4 Posterior superior iliac spine	10 Greater trochanter
	11 Shaft of femur
5 Posterior inferior iliac spine	ABC, Bryant's triangle

8
7

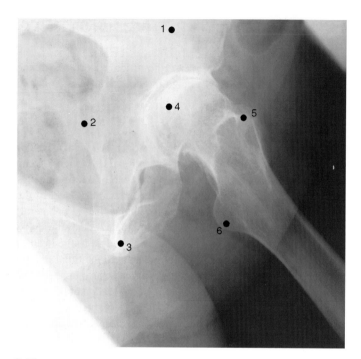

8.18
Hip joint: oblique view

1 Ilium
2 Ischial spine
3 Ischial tuberosity
4 Head of femur
5 Greater trochanter
6 Lesser trochanter

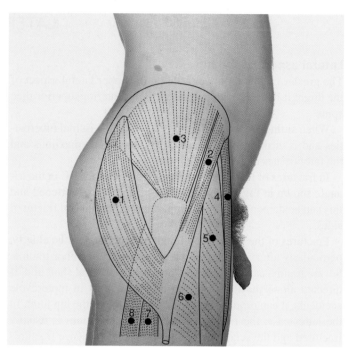

8.20
Lateral aspect of the hip joint: superficial muscles

1 Gluteus maximus
2 Tensor fascia lata
3 Gluteus medius
4 Sartorius
5 Rectus femoris
6 Vastus lateralis
7 Long head of biceps femoris
8 Semitendinosus

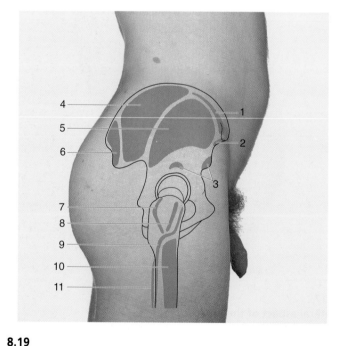

8.19
Lateral aspect of the hip joint: muscle attachments

1 Tensor fascia lata
2 Sartorius
3 Rectus femoris
4 and 7 Gluteus medius
5 and 8 Gluteus minimus
6 and 11 Gluteus maximus
9 Vastus lateralis
10 Vastus intermedius

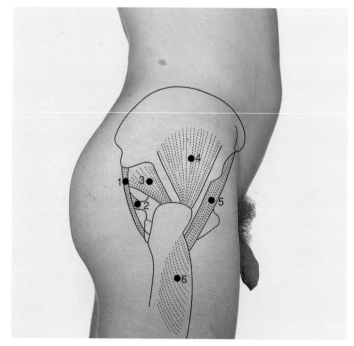

8.21
Lateral aspect of the hip joint: deep muscles and ligaments

1 Sacrotuberous ligament
2 Sacrospinous ligament
3 Piriformis
4 Gluteus minimus
5 Iliopsoas
6 Vastus lateralis

8

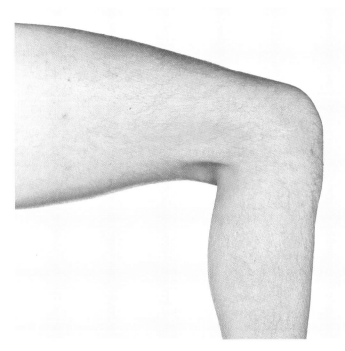

8.22
Lateral aspect of the flexed knee

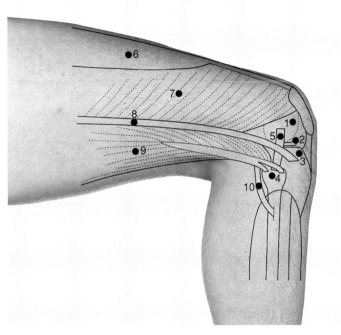

8.24
Lateral aspect of the flexed knee: bones and soft tissues

1 Lateral femoral condyle	6 Rectus femoris
2 Lateral meniscus	7 Vastus lateralis
3 Lateral tibial condyle	8 Iliotibial tract
4 Head of fibula	9 Biceps femoris
5 Lateral collateral ligament	10 Common peroneal nerve

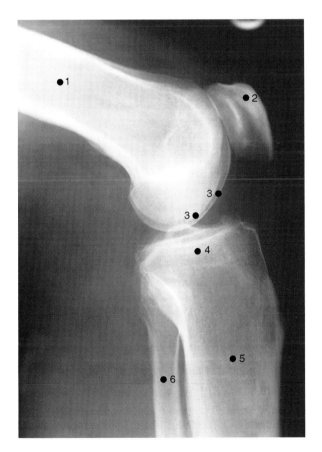

8.23
Knee: lateral view

1 Femoral shaft	4 Tibial condyle
2 Patella	5 Shaft of tibia
3 Femoral condyles	6 Shaft of fibula

8

POSTERIOR ASPECT OF THE HIP, THIGH AND KNEE

Gluteal region (Figs 8.19–8.21, 8.25–8.28)

The prominence of the buttock is formed from a large quadrilateral muscle, the gluteus maximus, covered by a variable, thick and even more extensive layer of fibrofatty superficial fascia. The muscle has an extensive proximal attachment, including the lateral surface of the ilium behind the posterior gluteal line, the sacrum, the coccyx and the sacrotuberous ligament. Fibres pass downwards and laterally to the iliotibial tract and the gluteal tuberosity on the femur. The muscle is a powerful lateral rotator and extensor of the hip joint and, through the iliotibial tract, it extends and stabilises the knee joint. The lower border of gluteus maximus does *not* correspond to the horizontal gluteal fold; the latter is the 'extensor line' or posterior skin fold, associated with the hip joint.

Gluteus maximus is supplied by the inferior gluteal nerve. The muscle overlies the hip joint and short articular muscles and the nerves, passing through the greater and lesser sciatic foramina, in particular the sciatic, gluteal and pudendal nerves. Injections into the buttock must be placed in the upper outer quadrant to avoid damage to these deep structures. The tensor fasciae lata is attached to the anterior quarter of the outer lip below the crest of the ilium and is distally attached to the iliotibial tract, acting with gluteus maximus, and stabilising and extending the knee joint. It is supplied by the superior gluteal nerve.

When standing on one leg, the non-weight-bearing side of the pelvis is raised to keep the non-weight-bearing leg off the ground. This action is brought about by the gluteus medius and minimus muscles attached to the anterolateral aspect of the ilium medially, and the greater trochanter laterally. They are supplied by the superior gluteal nerve and may be felt contracting through the gluteus maximus in this position.

Posterior aspect of the thigh

The muscle bulk of the posterior aspect of the thigh is formed from the hamstring muscles arising from the ischial tuberosity (Fig. 8.28). The semimembranosus is attached distally to a groove on the posteromedial aspect of the tibial condyle; and also by a tendinous expansion to the lateral femoral condyle (oblique popliteal ligament) and downwards to the soleal line of the tibia, forming the popliteal fascia over the popliteus muscle. Semitendinosus is attached distally to the upper subcutaneous

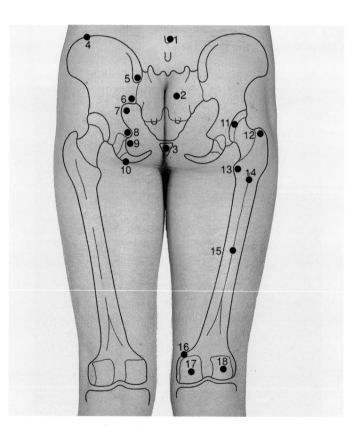

8.26
Gluteal region and posterior aspect of the thigh: bones

1 Fourth lumbar spine	9 Lesser sciatic notch
2 Sacrum	10 Ischial tuberosity
3 Coccyx	11 Head of femur
4 Iliac crest	12 Greater trochanter
5 Posterior superior iliac spine	13 Lesser trochanter
6 Posterior inferior iliac spine	14 Gluteal tuberosity
7 Greater sciatic notch	15 Linea aspera
8 Ischial spine	16 Adductor tubercle
	17 Medial femoral condyle
	18 Lateral femoral condyle

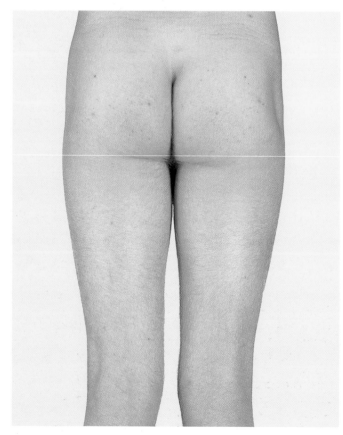

8.25
Gluteal region and posterior aspect of the thigh

medial surface of the tibia and the biceps to the head of the fibula; the latter muscle receives an additional short head from the linea aspera. The hamstring muscles are powerful extensors of the hip joint and flexors of the knee joint; they are supplied by the sciatic nerve. The biceps (laterally) and the semimembranosus and semitendinosus (medially) form an inverted V bordering the upper part of the popliteal fossa.

The sciatic nerve leaves the pelvis through the greater sciatic foramen and is related to the ischium and the small posterior articular muscles of the hip joint. It passes deep to the gluteus maximus and then the hamstring muscles before dividing into tibial and common peroneal terminal branches.

It may be damaged in posterior dislocation of the hip joint because of its close relation to the joint.

Popliteal fossa (Fig. 8.31)
The popliteal fossa is a diamond-shaped space behind the knee joint. The upper palpable margins are formed by the hamstring tendons and the lower margins by the medial and lateral heads of the gastrocnemius muscle. The fossa is roofed by the popliteal fascia, a thickening of the fascia lata; the floor is formed, from above downwards, by the posterior surface of the femur, the knee joint and the popliteus muscle over the upper tibia.

The fossa contains the popliteal vessels and the tibial and common peroneal nerves, fat and a few lymph nodes. The popliteal artery is deep to its vein and closely applied to the knee joint. It can be felt by deep compression along the length of the fossa, but most easily with the knee slightly flexed over the upper tibia.

Movements of the knee joint
The movements of the knee joint are flexion, extension and a little rotation. Flexion is by the hamstring muscles aided by gastrocnemius and limited by the approximation of the calf and thigh. Extension is by the quadriceps and the iliotibial tract muscles. The femoral condyles roll and also glide backwards on the tibial condyles until the cruciate ligaments become taut. Further extension (hyperextension) is brought about by medial rotation of the femur on the tibia around a taut anterior cruciate ligament.

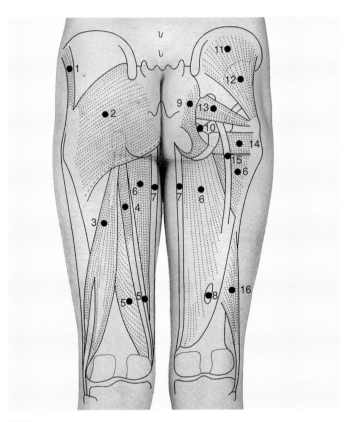

8.27
Gluteal region and posterior aspect of the thigh: muscle attachments

1 Gluteus medius	8 Adductor longus
2 Hamstring muscles	9 Short head of biceps femoris
3 Gluteus maximus	10 Vastus medialis
4 Iliopsoas	11 Adductor magnus
5 Pectineus	12 and 13 Gastrocnemius
6 Vastus lateralis	
7 Adductor brevis	

8.28
Gluteal region and posterior aspect of the thigh: superficial (left limb) and deep (right limb) muscles

1 Tensor fascia lata	10 Sacrospinous ligament
2 Gluteus maximus	11 Gluteus medius
3 Long head of biceps femoris	12 Gluteus minimus (deep to medius)
4 Semitendinosus	13 Piriformis
5 Semimembranosus	14 Quadratus femoris
6 Adductor magnus	15 Sciatic nerve
7 Gracilis	16 Short head of biceps femoris
8 Adductor hiatus	
9 Sacrotuberous ligament	

8

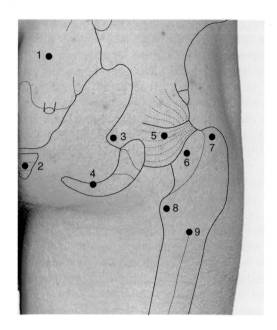

8.29
Hip joint: posterior aspect

1 Sacrum
2 Coccyx
3 Ischial spine
4 Ischial tuberosity
5 Ischiofemoral ligament
6 Femur
7 Greater trochanter
8 Lesser trochanter
9 Gluteal tuberosity

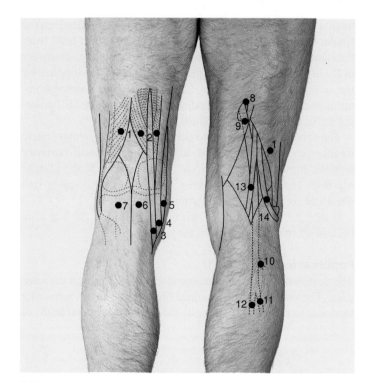

8.31
Popliteal fossa: soft tissues
(For the sake of clarity, the popliteal vein, which descends between the popliteal artery and the tibial nerve, has been omitted)

1 Biceps femoris
2 Semimembranosus
3 Semitendinosus
4 Gracilis
5 Sartorius
6 Gastrocnemius, medial head
7 Gastrocnemius, lateral head
8 Adductor hiatus
9 Popliteal artery
10 Anterior tibial artery
11 Peroneal artery
12 Posterior tibial artery
13 Tibial nerve
14 Common peroneal nerve

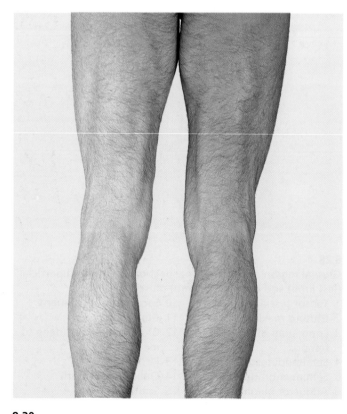

8.30
Popliteal fossa

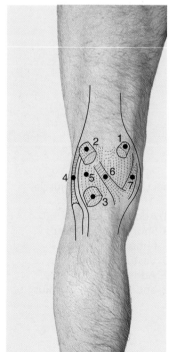

8.32
Knee joint: posterior aspect

1 and 2 Gastrocnemius
3 Popliteus
4 Lateral ligament
5 Posterior capsule
6 Oblique popliteal ligament
7 Medial ligament

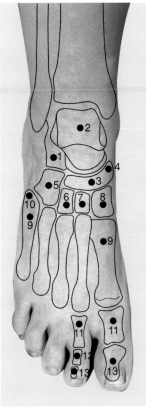

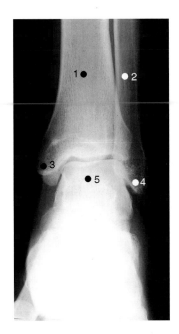

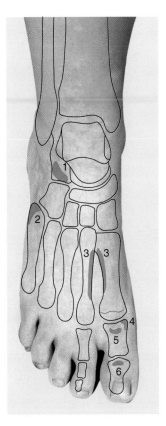

8.39
Ankle: anterior view
1 Shaft of tibia
2 Shaft of fibula
3 Medial malleolus
4 Lateral malleolus;
5 Talus

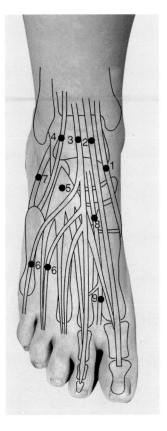

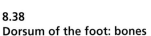

8.38
Dorsum of the foot: bones
1 Calcaneus
2 Talus
3 Navicular
4 Tubercle of navicular bone
5 Cuboid
6 Lateral cuneiform
7 Intermediate cuneiform
8 Medial cuneiform
9 Metatarsals
10 Tuberosity (styloid) of fifth metatarsal bone
11 Proximal phalanges
12 Middle phalanges
13 Distal phalanges

8.40
Dorsum of the foot: muscle attachments
1 Extensor digitorum brevis
2 Peroneus brevis
3 First dorsal interosseus
4 Abductor hallucis
5 Extensor hallucis brevis
6 Extensor hallucis longus

8.41
Dorsum of the foot: tendons
1 Tibialis anterior
2 Extensor hallucis longus
3 Extensor digitorum longus
4 Peroneus tertius
5 Extensor digitorum brevis
6 Extensor tendons
7 Peroneus brevis
8 Dorsalis pedis artery
9 First dorsal metatarsal artery

MEDIAL ASPECT OF THE LOWER LEG

The medial surface of the tibia is subcutaneous throughout its length and is prone to trauma, ranging from superficial cuts to fractures of the bone. The lower end of the bone is expanded into the medial malleolus, articulating with the talus on its lateral side (Fig. 8.43). The posterior medial aspect of the calcaneus, the sustentaculum tali, the tubercle of the navicular, and the medial aspect of the first metatarsal and its two phalanges are palpable along the medial aspect of the foot (for relative positions see Figs 8.42, 8.43).

The sartorius, gracilis and semitendinosus muscles are attached to the upper subcutaneous surface of the tibia. The tendons of the deep posterior muscles of the calf groove the lower end of the tibia; these are not all palpable but the tibialis posterior, and flexor digitorum longus lateral to it, can be felt just above and medial to the posterior tibial artery. The surface marking of the artery at the ankle joint is between the prominence of the medial malleolus and the medial prominence of the calcaneus. It can be palpated by compression on the talus before it passes deeply into the sole. The deep tendons are covered by a deep thickening in the fascia, the flexor retinaculum; it passes between the medial malleolus and the medial tubercle of the calcaneus. Each tendon has a separate sheath deep to the retinaculum.

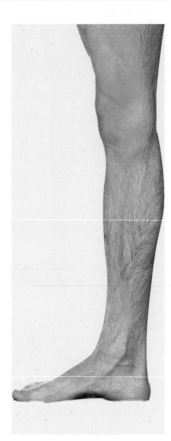

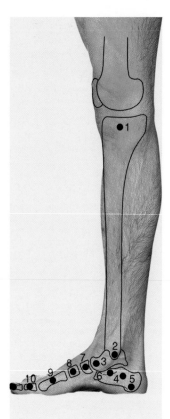

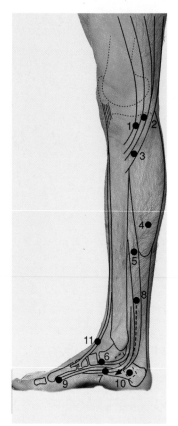

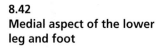

8.45
Ankle joint: medial aspect
1 Medial ligament
2 Posterior tibiotalar
   ligament
3 Anterior ligament
4 Plantar calcaneonavicular
   ligament
5 Long plantar ligament

8.42
**Medial aspect of the lower
leg and foot**

8.43
**Medial aspect of the lower
leg and foot: bones**
   1 Tibia
   2 Medial malleolus
   3 Talus
   4 Calcaneus
   5 Medial tubercle of
     calcaneus
   6 Sustentaculum tali
   7 Navicular (tubercle)
   8 Medial cuneiform
   9 First metatarsal
  10 Phalanges

8.44
**Medial aspect of the lower
leg and foot: muscles**
   1 Sartorius
   2 Gracilis
   3 Semitendinosus
   4 Gastrocnemius
   5 Soleus
   6 Tibialis posterior
   7 Flexor digitorum longus
   8 Posterior tibial artery
     (dotted)
   9 Flexor hallucis longus
  10 Flexor retinaculum
  11 Tibialis anterior

On deep pressure about 2 cm below the tip of the medial malleolus, the sustentaculum tali can be felt and is a good clinical landmark for the tendons. Tibialis posterior curves downwards and forwards above the sustentaculum; flexor digitorum longus crosses its medial surface, sometimes grooving it; flexor hallucis longus lies in a deep groove on the inferior aspect (below) of the sustentaculum.

LATERAL ASPECT OF THE LOWER LEG

The head of the fibula is palpable below the knee joint but its shaft is surrounded by muscle bellies. The lower end of the bone is expanded into the lateral malleolus; this is 1 cm lower than the medial and contributes to the mortise of the ankle joint. The lateral surface of the calcaneus, its peroneal tubercle, the cuboid and the tuberosity (styloid) of the base of the fifth metatarsal are readily palpable along this surface (Fig. 8.47). The two lateral (evertor) compartment muscles are the peroneus longus and peroneus brevis, attached respectively to the upper two-thirds and lower third of the lateral surface of the fibula (Fig. 8.49). The palpable tendons pass behind the lateral malleolus (the peroneus brevis muscle and tendon are anterior) and cross the lateral surface of the calcaneus, above (brevis) and below (longus) the peroneal tubercle.

The peroneus longus tendon grooves the under surface of the cuboid and is attached to the base of the first metatarsal and adjacent medial cuneiform bone. The tendon of the peroneus brevis passes to the tuberosity of the base of the fifth metatarsal bone. The two muscles evert and plantarflex the foot; they are supplied by the superficial peroneal nerve. The tendons are bound down to the lateral malleolus and calcaneus by two thickenings in the deep fascia, the superior and inferior peroneal retinaculae. The tendons are enclosed in a common synovial sheath which is prolonged over each to its distal attachment.

Lower leg fractures usually involve both the tibia and fibula and, in view of the subcutaneous position of the tibia, these fractures are usually compound (i.e. open to the air, through the intervening skin laceration).

Rotational injuries of the ankle are common and usually involve the lateral and medial ligaments. In more severe injuries, the lateral and medial malleoli may be fractured, and in major trauma, the posterior rim of the tibia (posterior malleolus) is also fractured, and the ankle joint dislocated.

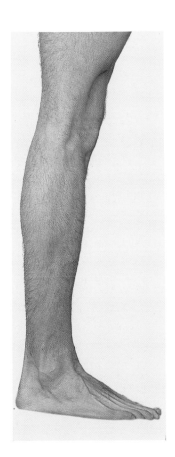
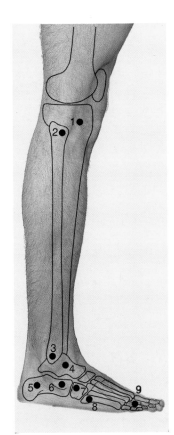
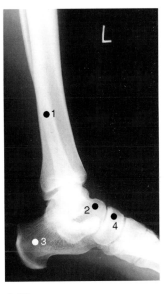

8.47
Lateral aspect of the lower leg and foot: bones
1 Tibia
2 Head of fibula
3 Lateral malleolus
4 Talus
5 Calcaneus
6 Peroneal tubercle of calcaneus
7 Cuboid
8 Fifth metatarsal
9 Phalanges

8.48
Ankle: lateral view
1 Overlapping shafts of tibia and fibula
2 Talus
3 Calcaneus
4 Navicular

8.46
Lateral aspect of the lower leg and foot

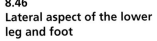

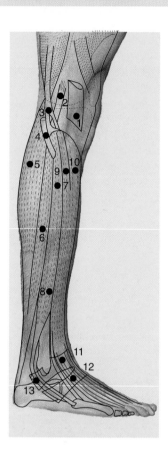

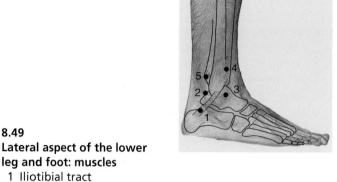

8.50
Ankle joint: lateral aspect
1 Calcaneofibular ligament
2 Posterior talofibular ligament
3 Anterior talofibular ligament
4 Anterior tibiofibular ligament
5 Posterior tibiofibular ligament

8.49
Lateral aspect of the lower leg and foot: muscles
1 Iliotibial tract
2 Lateral collateral ligament
3 Biceps femoris tendon
4 Common peroneal nerve
5 Gastrocnemius
6 Soleus
7 Peroneus longus
8 Peroneus brevis
9 Extensor digitorum longus
10 Tibialis anterior
11 and 13 Superior extensor retinaculum
12 Inferior extensor retinaculum

POSTERIOR ASPECT OF THE LOWER LEG

The bulk of the calf is formed of the gastrocnemius and soleus muscles which unite inferiorly to form the tendo calcaneus to be attached to the middle of the posterior surface of the calcaneus (Fig. 8.54). A bursa and a pad of fat separate the tendon from the upper posterior calcaneal surface. The gastrocnemius is superficial to the soleus and it has medial and lateral

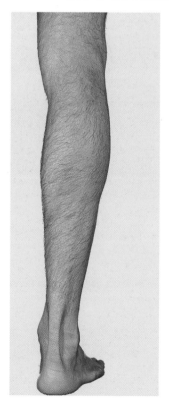

8.51
Posterior aspect of the lower leg and heel

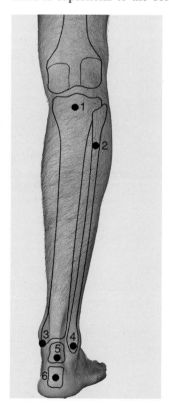

8.52
Posterior aspect of the lower leg and heel: bones
1 Tibia
2 Fibula
3 Medial malleolus
4 Lateral malleolus
5 Talus
6 Calcaneus

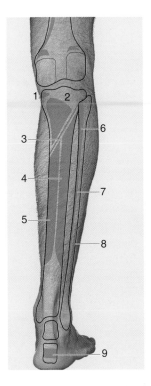

8.53
Posterior aspect of the lower leg and heel: muscle attachments
1 Semimembranosus
2 Popliteus
3 and 6 Soleus
4 Tibialis posterior
5 Flexor digitorum longus
7 Flexor hallucis longus
8 Peroneus brevis
9 Tendo calcaneus

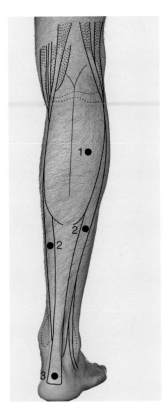

8.54
Posterior aspect of the lower leg and heel: superficial muscles
1 Gastrocnemius
2 Soleus
3 Tendo calcaneus

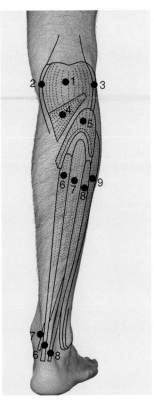

8.55
Posterior aspect of the lower leg and heel: deep muscles
1 Capsule of knee joint
2 Tibial collateral ligament
3 Fibular collateral ligament
4 Popliteus
5 Soleus – partly excised
6 Flexor digitorum longus
7 Tibialis posterior
8 Flexor hallucis longus
9 Peroneal muscles

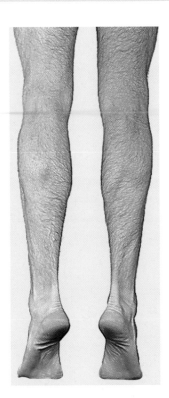

8.56
Posterior aspect of the leg when standing on the toes

heads attached to the respective femoral condyles. The soleus has a continuous upper attachment from the head of the fibula, a tendinous arch over the posterior tibial vessels and tibial nerve, and to the soleal line on the tibia. It bulges out on either side of the gastrocnemius in the calf. These muscles are powerful plantar flexors of the foot and are important in both posture and locomotion; they are supplied by the tibial nerve. Within and between the muscles is a plexus of veins, and contraction of the muscles expels blood proximally (the muscle pump). The plantaris is a thin vestigial muscle along the lateral head of the gastrocnemius. The deep muscles of the calf are impalpable above the ankle region.

8

SOLE OF THE FOOT

The skin over the weight-bearing areas of the heel and the ball of the foot is thick and firmly attached to the fascia and its thickened central plantar aponeurosis by fibrous septa. These septa loculate subcutaneous fat producing a cushioning effect over the underlying tissues. The posterior aspect of the calcaneus and the heads of the metatarsals are palpable through this cushion but the remaining bones are deep to the short muscles (Fig. 8.58). A sesamoid bone, embedded in the short tendons, is present on each side of the head of the first metatarsal.

The pattern of the small muscles of the foot is similar to that of the hand, but there are no opponens muscles and the flexor accessorius has no upper limb counterpart. The latter muscle is attached to the calcaneus posteriorly and to the lateral aspect of the tendon of the flexor digitorum longus anteriorly. The medial

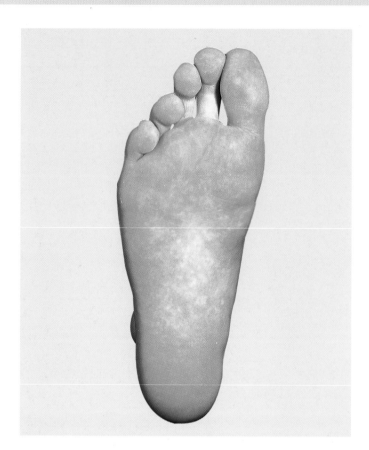

8.57
Sole of the foot

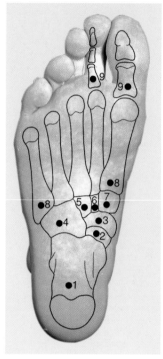

8.58
Sole of the foot: bones
1 Calcaneus
2 Talus
3 Navicular
4 Cuboid
5 Lateral cuneiform
6 Intermediate cuneiform
7 Medial cuneiform
8 Metatarsals
9 Phalanges

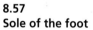

planter nerve supplies abductor hallucis, flexor hallicus brevis, flexor digitorum brevis and the first lumbrical; the remaining muscles are supplied by the lateral plantar nerve (Fig. 8.60). The long flexor tendons pass through the sole to gain attachment to the distal phalanges, flexing the toes, assisted by small muscles which also can produce slight fanning of the toes. The tendon of tibialis posterior passes to the tuberosity of the navicular and gives slips to most other tarsal and metatarsal bones.

The small muscles act with the long flexor tendons to maintain the plantar arches. These provide resilience to the foot and distribute the body weight over the sole, while still allowing it to act as a semi-rigid lever propelling the body forwards. The arches can be divided into medial and lateral longitudinal, and transverse, but they act as a single unit. Each arch is maintained by bony, ligamentous and muscular factors.

The medial longitudinal arch is formed of the calcaneus, talus, navicular, three cuneiform and three medial metatarsal bones. The sustentaculum tali of the calcaneus gives support to the head of the talus and there is also some wedging of the bones along the length of the arch aiding its support. The plantar calcaneonavicular (spring) ligament supports the head of the talus and further contributions are from strong interosseous ligaments. The plantar aponeurosis ties the ends of the arch together, as do the long flexors of the hallux and adjacent two toes, with contributions from the short medial muscles of the sole. The tibialis anterior muscle provides powerful support from its attachments to the centre of the arch.

The lateral longitudinal arch is lower than the medial and is formed of the calcaneus, cuboid and fourth and fifth metatarsal bones; it is maintained mainly by ligaments, in particular the long and short plantars. The tendon of peroneus longus is beneath the centre of the arch and the long and short digital muscles provide some support. The transverse arch is maintained mainly by the wedge-shaped nature of the cuboid and cuneiform bones and their strong interosseous ligaments. The attachments of the peroneus longus and tibialis posterior provide some muscular support.

8

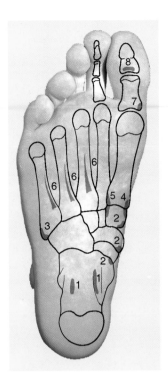

8.59
Sole of the foot: muscle attachments
1 Flexor digitorum accessorius
2 Tibialis posterior
3 Peroneus brevis
4 Tibialis anterior
5 Peroneus longus
6 Plantar interossei
7 Abductor hallucis
8 Flexor hallucis longus

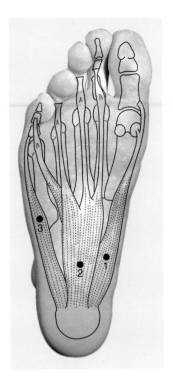

8.60
Sole of the foot: plantar fascia
1 Plantar aponeurosis
2 Transverse bands
3 Digital bands
4 Superficial transverse metacarpal ligament

8.61
Sole of the foot: first muscle layer
1 Abductor digiti minimi
2 Flexor digitorum brevis
3 Abductor hallucis

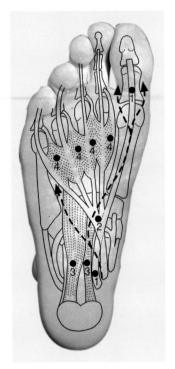

8.62
Sole of the foot: second muscle layer
1 Flexor hallucis longus
2 Flexor digitorum longus
3 Flexor digitorum accessorius
4 Four lumbrical muscles

The dotted line indicates the position of the posterior tibial artery and the tibial nerve. On entering the foot they divide into medial and lateral plantar vessels and nerves

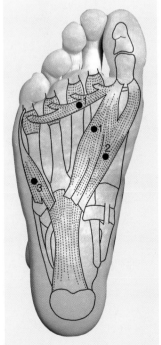

8.63
Sole of the foot: third muscle layer
1 Adductor hallucis
2 Flexor hallucis brevis
3 Flexor digiti minimi brevis

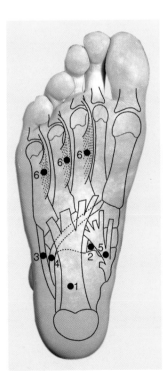

8.64
Sole of the foot: fourth muscle layer
1 Long plantar ligament
2 Plantar calcaneonavicular ligament
3 Peroneus brevis
4 Peroneus longus
5 Tibialis posterior
6 Plantar interossei

8

MOVEMENTS OF THE ANKLE AND INTERTARSAL JOINTS

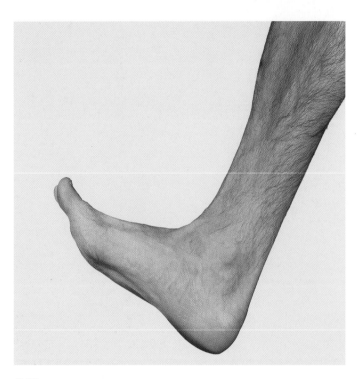

8.65
Dorsiflexion of the foot

The ankle joint is a hinge joint between the talus and the mortise, formed between the lower ends of the tibia and fibula. The shape of the bones and powerful interosseous and medial and lateral ligaments maintain the stability of the joint. It is least stable in the plantarflexed position. Dorsiflexion is produced by tibialis anterior and other muscles of the extensor compartment of the leg; plantarflexion is primarily by the gastrocnemius and soleus muscles.

The subtalar (posterior talocalcaneal) and talocalcaneonavicular joints act as a single unit at which inversion and eversion take place. Inversion (turning the sole inwards) is produced by tibialis anterior and posterior, and limited by tension in the peroneus longus and brevis muscles, and the interosseous talocalcaneal ligament. The movement is increased in plantarflexion and by movement at the midtarsal (talonavicular and calcaneocuboid) joint. Eversion (turning the sole outwards) is produced by the peroneal muscles and limited by the tibialis anterior and posterior muscles, and the medial ligament of the ankle joint. The movement is increased in dorsiflexion and by movement at the midtarsal joint. These movements are described with the foot off the ground; the same movements with the foot on the ground adjust the foot and lower limb to uneven and sloping surfaces. Also, when the foot is weight-bearing, there are additional movements of supination and pronation of the distal tarsus and metatarsus (forefoot) relative to the talus and calcaneus (hindfoot).

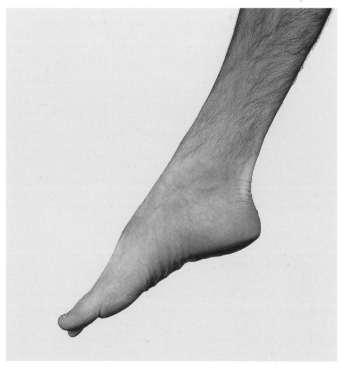

8.66
Plantarflexion of the foot

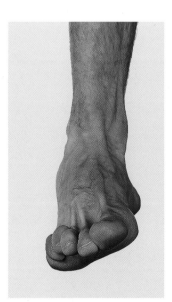

8.67
Inversion of the foot

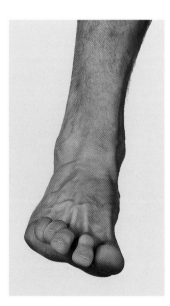

8.68
Eversion of the foot

INNERVATION OF THE LOWER LIMB

The lower limb is innervated by the sacral plexus. The groin gains additional sensory contributions from L1 and the perineal region from S3. Note that one kneels on L3 and L4, walks on S1 and sits on S3. The knee jerk is supplied by L3 and L4, the ankle jerk by S1 and the plantar reflex by S1 and S2. The L5 root is not represented in these reflexes but can be specifically tested in dorsiflexion of the great toe.

Injury to the femoral nerve produces loss of knee extension (quadriceps), some loss of hip flexion (iliacus and pectineus) and loss of sensation of the front and medial side of the thigh, leg and foot (anterior and medial femoral cutaneous, and the saphenous nerves). Damage to the obturator nerve denervates the adductor muscles but some adduction is retained because of the sciatic contribution to the adductor magnus; often there is no sensory loss.

The sciatic nerve may be injured in posterior dislocation of the hip joint: this produces an almost flail limb. A distal injury may spare the branches to the hamstrings and allow knee flexion. Injury to the tibial nerve produces loss of plantarflexion and sensory denervation of the sole of the foot.

Injury to the tibial nerve, near the ankle, denervates the small muscles of the sole; the unopposed action of the long flexor and extensor muscles produces a highly arched foot. Injury proximal to the origin of the sural nerve also produces loss of sensation of the lateral side of the leg and foot.

The common peroneal nerve is the most commonly injured nerve in the leg. This is often associated with fractures of the neck of the fibula or a badly fitting leg plaster. The power of dorsiflexion (extensor muscles) and eversion (peroneal muscles) is lost, and the foot drops and becomes inverted: there is sensory loss over the medial side of the dorsum of the foot. In superficial peroneal nerve injuries, the foot is inverted due to loss of eversion (peronei): sensory loss is over the medial part of the dorsum of the foot. In deep peroneal nerve injuries, the power of dorsiflexion of the foot and toes is lost and there may be loss of sensation between the first and second toes: the foot becomes inverted by the unopposed action of the tibialis posterior muscle.

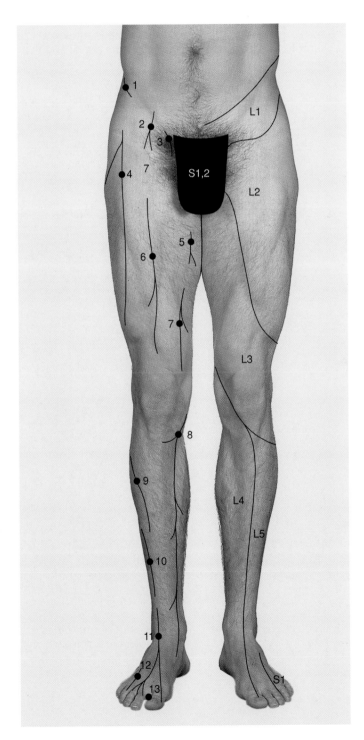

8.69
Cutaneous nerves and dermatomes of the lower limb: anterior

1 12th thoracic
2 Femoral branch of genitofemoral
3 Ilioinguinal
4 Lateral cutaneous nerve of thigh
5 Obturator
6 Intermediate femoral cutaneous
7 Medial cutaneous nerve of thigh
8 Saphenous
9 Lateral cutaneous nerve of leg
10 Musculocutaneous
11 Superficial peroneal
12 Sural
13 Anterior tibial

L, Lumbar
S, Sacral

The numbers on the left limb, scrotum and perineum denote the nerve roots

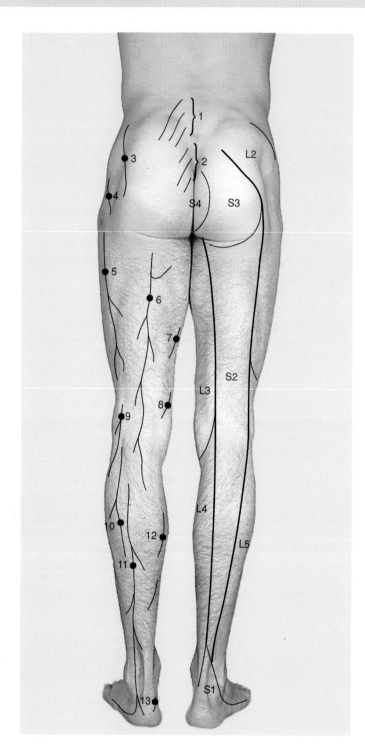

8.70
Cutaneous nerves and dermatomes of the lower limb: posterior

1 Lumbar
2 Sacral
3 Iliohypogastric
4 12th thoracic
5 Lateral cutaneous nerve of thigh
6 Posterior cutaneous nerve of thigh
7 Obturator
8 Medial cutaneous nerve of thigh

9 Lateral cutaneous nerve of calf
10 Sural communicating
11 Sural
12 Saphenous
13 Tibial

L, Lumbar
S, Sacral

The numbers on the right limb denote lumbar and sacral nerve roots. The bold right line indicates the dorsal and the left the ventral axial lines

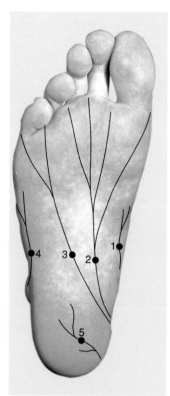

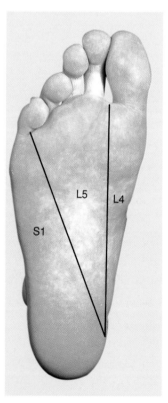

8.71
Cutaneous innervation of the sole
1 Saphenous
2 Medial plantar
3 Lateral plantar
4 Sural
5 Tibial

8.72
Cutaneous dermatomes of the sole: lumbar fourth and fifth and first sacral nerve roots

8

VESSELS OF THE LOWER LIMB

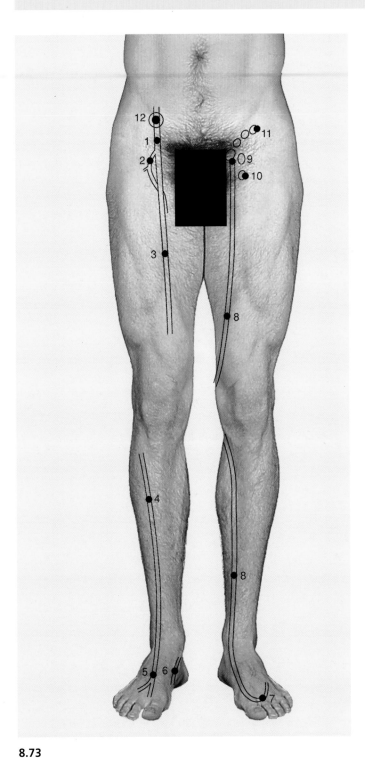

8.73
Vessels of the lower limb: anterior

1 Femoral (common femoral) artery
2 Deep femoral artery
3 Femoral (superficial femoral) artery
4 Anterior tibial artery
5 Dorsalis pedis artery
6 Posterior tibial artery
7 Dorsal venous arch
8 Great saphenous vein
9 Saphenous opening (see also Fig. 8.7)
10 Vertical chain of inguinal lymph nodes
11 Horizontal chain of inguinal lymph nodes
12 Point of access to femoral artery

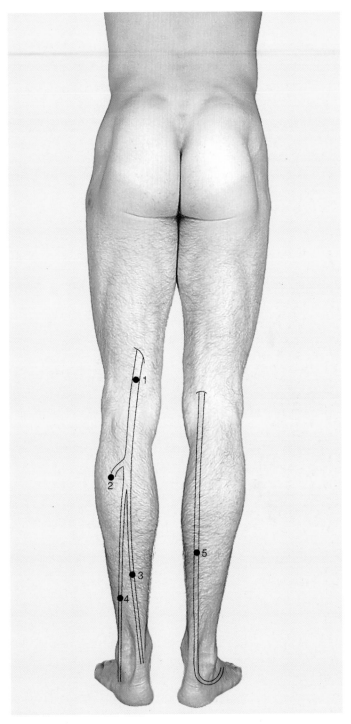

8.74
Vessels of the lower limb: posterior

1 Popliteal artery
2 Anterior tibial artery
3 Posterior tibial artery
4 Peroneal artery
5 Small saphenous vein

8

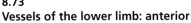

9 ACUPUNCTURE

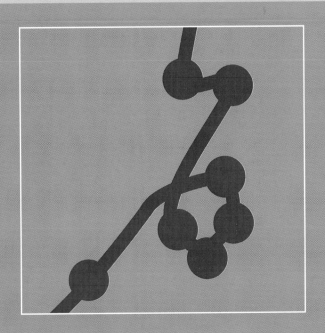

Acupuncture is a traditional form of Chinese medicine that has existed for more than 5000 years. It provides care for a quarter of the world's population. After the Chinese Cultural Revolution, more than a million barefoot doctors were trained in the technique, applying these skills in industrial and rural communities in a safe, simple, effective and economical way throughout China. Acupuncture presents a possible long- as well as short-term answer to the health care needs of populations across a large part of the Asian subcontinent; it is also practised in many centres in the Western world.

The technique is based on the finding that manipulation of the surface of the body can alleviate disease and suffering. Widely separated points were found to have similar therapeutic properties, and these series of acupuncture points were termed 'channels' or 'meridians'. Initially, needles were made of stone, but they gradually evolved through bone and bamboo to their current metal form.

ACUPUNCTURE CHANNELS

There are 12 regular and eight extraordinary channels, and vital energy (Qi) is considered to flow along them. The 12 regular channels are each linked to an internal organ. Of these, six are 'solid' and termed *Zang organs* (Chinese: to store) and six are 'hollow' and termed *Fu organs* (Chinese: to receive). Zang organs are the lung (Lu), spleen (Sp), heart (H), kidney (K), pericardium (P) and liver (Liv), and Fu organs are the large intestine (LI), stomach (St), small intestine (SI), urinary bladder (UB), sanjiao (SJ – the three body cavities, also called the triple-warmer and triple energiser) and gall bladder (GB). The channels are named after the organs with which they are linked.

The channel–organ combinations are called *Yin* (Zang organs) or *Yang* (Fu organs). The six Zang and six Fu organs are coupled (Lu : LI, Sp : St, H : SI, K : UB, P : SJ, Liv : GB) and because of this, the Yin and Yang channels are referred to as the '12 paired channels' (they are also referred to as organ or visceral channels). Although Zang and Fu organs have different sets of functions, their interrelation preserves the unity and integrity of the organism and maintains the balance of vital functions.

Of the eight extraordinary channels, two run in the midline: the *Ren channel* (Chinese: the front) along the anterior trunk, and the *Du channel* (Chinese: the governor) along the back. Point 20 (Baihui) on the Du channel governs all other points and channels, hence the Du is often referred to as the *governor channel*.

The other six extraordinary channels do not have their own points, but are formed by interconnection between the points of the 12 paired and the two midline channels. Thus, 12 paired and two midline extraordinary channels have their own points, and they are collectively known as 'the 14 channels' – as shown in the subsequent illustrations. The 12 paired channels are bilaterally represented but only one side is illustrated in each case.

The normal level of vital energy (Qi) in a healthy individual is maintained by the balance of Yin and Yang factors. The ancient Chinese also postulated that Qi circulated (*Jing-Qi*) in the 12 paired channels in a set sequence (Fig. 9.1). Jing-Qi was thought to pass distally in the arm through the three Yin channels on the anterior aspect (Lu, H, P – 'the three Yin channels of the hand') and return through the three Yang channels on the posterior aspect (LI, SI, SJ – 'the three Yang channels of the hand'). The three circuits were completed by Jing-Qi passing distally in the leg through the three Yang channels on the anterior, posterior and lateral aspects (St, UB, GB – 'the three Yang channels of the foot'), returning through the three Yin channels on the medial aspect (Sp, K, Liv – 'the three Yin channels of the foot'). The sequence of the three cycles was thus: Lu, LI, St, Sp; H, SI, UB, K; P, SJ, GB, Liv; the illustrations follow this order (Figs 9.2–9.13).

Disease, exogenous factors (such as heat, cold, wind, fire) and endogenous factors (such as joy, anger, melancholy, shock) produce imbalance of the Qi within the body. The prime objective

9.1
Flow of vital energy in the 12 paired channels

9

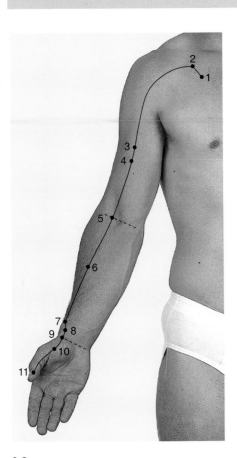

9.2
Lung channel – Lu

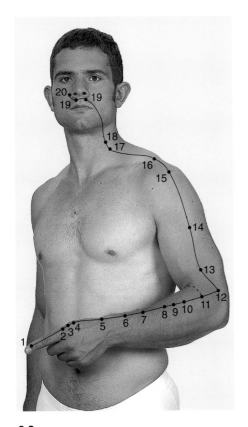

9.3
Large intestine channel – LI

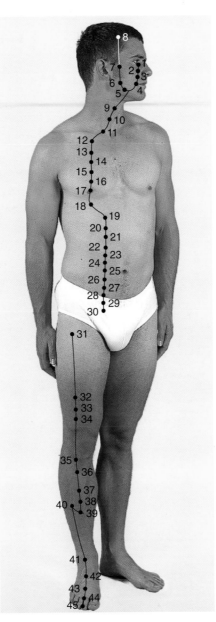

9.4
Stomach channel – St

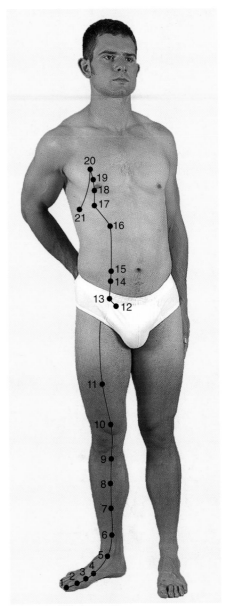

9.5
Spleen channel – Sp

Key to nomenclature for the 14 channels

Channel	Alphabetic code	
	Contemporary	Former
Lung	LU	Lu, P
Large intestine	LI	CO, Co, IC
Stomach	ST	S, St, E, M
Spleen	SP	Sp, LP
Heart	HT	H, C, Ht, He
Small intestine	SI	Si, IT
Bladder	BL	B, Bi, UB
Kidney	KI	Ki, R, Rn, K
Pericardium	PC	P, Pe, HC
Sanjiao (triple energiser)	TE	T, TW, SJ, 3H, TB
Gall bladder	GB	G, VB, VF
Liver	LR	Liv, LV, H
Du (governor vessel)	GV	Du, Go, Gv, TM
Ren (conception vessel)	CV	Co, Cv, J, REN, Ren

9

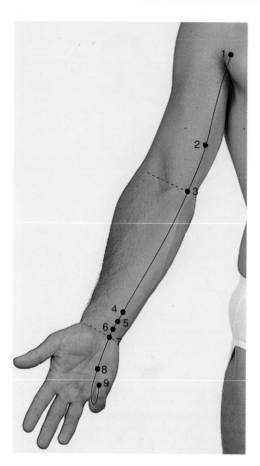

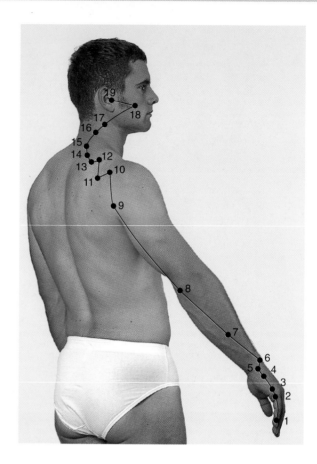

9.7
Small intestine channel – SI

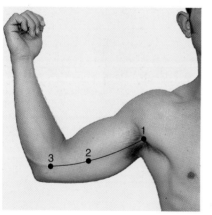

A

9.6
Heart channel – H (panel A: upper limb)

of acupuncture is to correct this imbalance by skilful manipulation at the surface level.

The concept of the internal organ in Chinese medicine is radically different from anatomical definitions used in the West. Although the Chinese terms are similar, they do not relate to a specific tissue, but rather to a series of closely interrelated functions, the main purpose of Chinese medicine being to diagnose the syndrome and institute specific treatment for the whole patient.

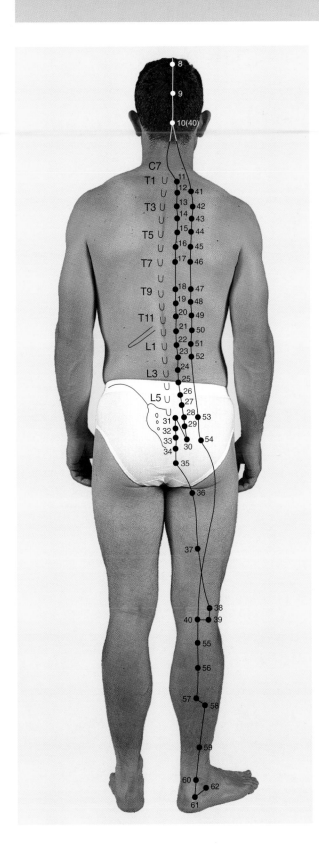

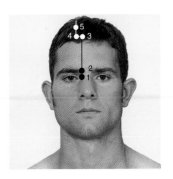

A

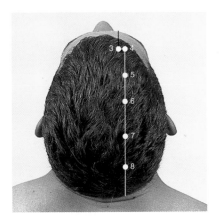

B

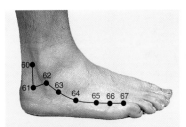

C

9.8
**Bladder channel – UB (panel A: face;
panel B: scalp; panel C: lateral foot)**

9

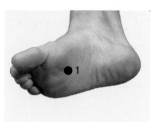

A

9.9
Kidney channel – K
(panel A: sole of foot)

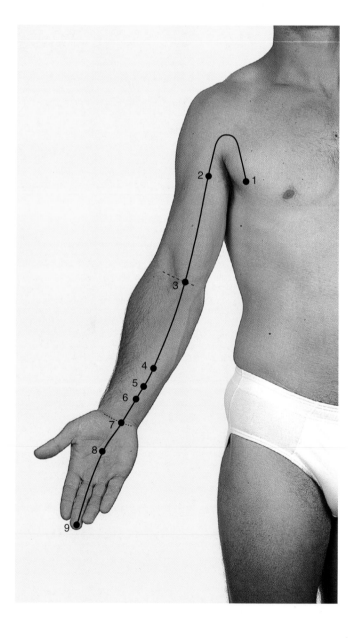

9.10
Pericardial channel – P

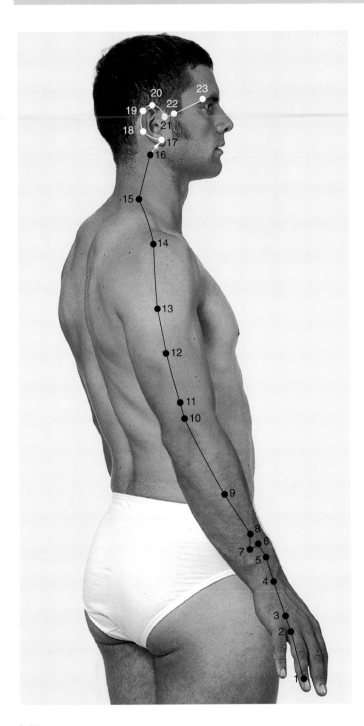

9.11
Sanjiao channel – SJ

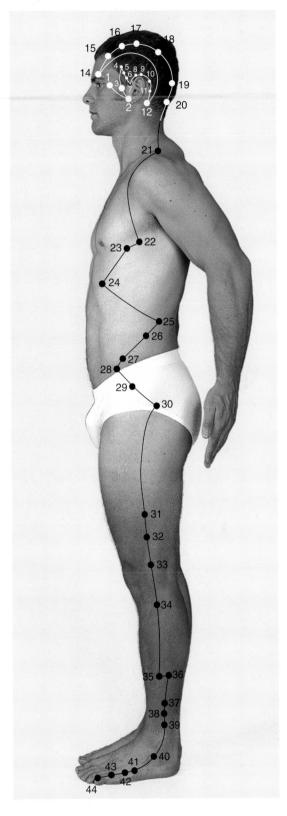

9.12
Gall bladder channel – GB

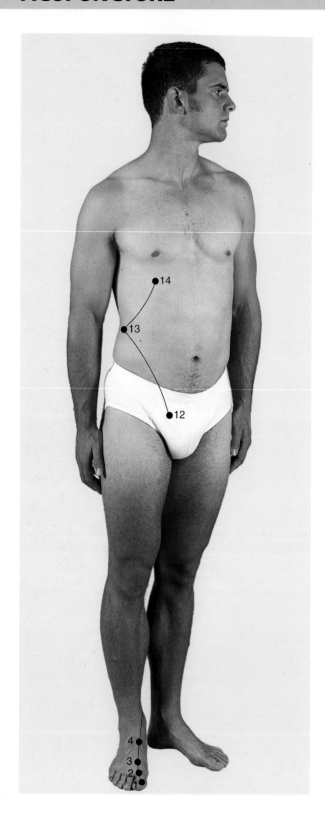

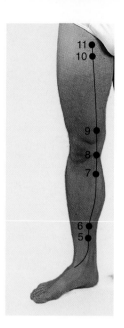

A

9.13
Liver channel – Liv (panel A: medial leg)

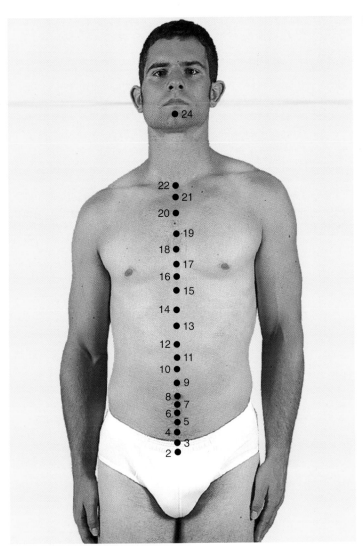

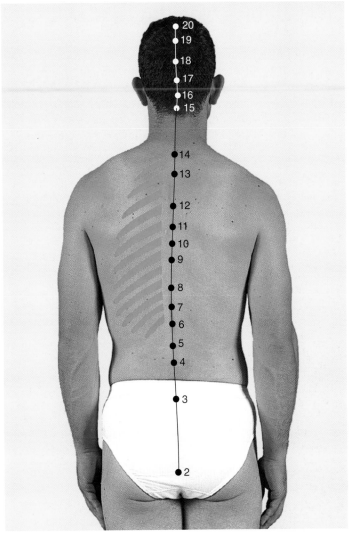

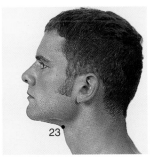

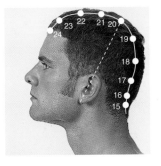

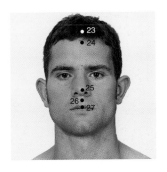

9.14
Ren channel – Ren
Ren 1 – in centre of perineum (panel A: lateral face)

A

A

B

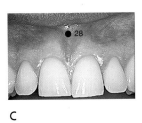

C

9.15
Du 1 – midway between coccyx and anus (panel A: side of head; panel B: face; panel C: lip)

9

IDENTIFYING ACUPUNCTURE POINTS

Identification of acupuncture points is primarily by palpation of anatomical landmarks, but for points situated some way from these landmarks, distances are measured in units (the *cun*) related to the subject's own stature. The cun is the maximum width of the thumb, or the distance between the creases over the proximal and distal interphalangeal joints of the middle finger, identified by opposing the tip of this finger to the thumb to form a circle. The breadth of the index and middle fingers is 1.5 cuns, and of all four fingers is 3 cuns. Other lengths relate to anatomical landmarks – for instance, in the midline, the anterior to posterior hairline is 12 cuns, and the anterior hairline to the brow is 3 cuns. The inter-nipple distance is 8 cuns, and the elbow to the wrist crease is 12 cuns. More sophisticated measures have used electrical conductivity, identifying acupuncture sites as points of lowered electrical resistance. When an acupuncture needle is accurately placed, the subject experiences a specific sensation (Deqi). This may be numbness, heaviness, soreness or distension, the specific feature depending on the chosen site of needling.

It is worthy of note that one non-traditional school maintains that acupuncture points do not exist, but rather that it is sufficient to needle the correct segment, dermatome or myotome.